Contents

Foreword

The MRCP is not an easy exam and nor should it be. Only the competent—and the dedicated—will pass. But it is possible to nudge the exam result in your favour if you prepare for it properly.

The format of the MRCP has changed several times over the years, but it has always contained theoretical and practical (clinical) elements. Passing the theoretical section of the exam is tough, but it equips you with the required knowledge to attempt the clinical section. Success depends upon making the best use of this hard-earned knowledge. The current clinical part of the MRCP–PACES is designed to be a fair and reproducible test, and has come as near as possible to the real world of patient care.

This book is designed to help you through the clinical stage of the MRCP. The important thing about it is that it has been written by experts—not the 'do as I say but not as I do' teachers, but by people who have recently gained their MRCP by actually doing PACES. The three authors wrote the book while Senior House Officers in medicine at Queen's Medical Centre, Nottingham; a busy teaching hospital with a high turnover of medical patients. This volume of practical experience shines through in their approach to PACES.

The QMC Senior House Officers are always a splendid group—intelligent, hardworking, full of common sense and (nearly always) cheerful, and working with them is one of the great pleasures of this hospital. The pass rate in the MRCP at QMC is often 100% and SHOs elsewhere will not do better than to learn from their contemporaries at QMC. They can do that by following the advice given in this book.

John Hampton
Professor of Cardiology, Queen's Medical Centre, Nottingham

Preface

PACES (Practical Assessment of Clinical Examination Skills), which was initiated in June 2001 by the Royal College of Physicians, has replaced the old style long case, short cases and viva format. The exam now comprises five stations in a carousel: History Taking (20 minutes), Communication Skills and Ethics (20 minutes), Cardiology/Neurology (10 minutes each), Respiratory/Abdominal (10 minutes each) and Short Cases (Skin, Locomotor, Eyes and Endocrine: 5 minutes each). The main changes are that candidates must take a history and communicate medical diagnoses to lay patients in front of their examiners. The viva is replaced by 'discussions' that occur at the end of each case, which concentrate on management issues relating to the case.

Cases for PACES mimics the new exam format, and is designed for use in an interactive way. It covers the new stations, with useful information on ethical and legal issues, history-taking advice and worked examples. It also provides mock questions for candidates to practise themselves.

Common cases rather than rarities have been deliberately chosen and are set out in an exam format. It is taken as read that candidates will be familiar in examination techniques and the appropriate order in which to elicit the various signs. In the book, only the key diagnostic clinical signs are documented, followed by extra points that will ensure you score high marks in the case. What follows in the discussion are some of the potential topics that a candidate could be expected to comment on at the end of the case, focusing particularly on management issues. The detail is not exhaustive but rather what is reasonably needed to pass. There is additional room for candidates to make further notes as they see fit. This book is designed to enable groups of candidates to practise 'under exam conditions' at the bedside.

The aim of this book is to put the information that is frequently tested in the clinical PACES exam in a succinct format that will enable capable candidates to pass with ease.

Good luck.

SH, AF, DH

Acknowledgements

We would like to thank Professor Peter Rubin, Dr David Seddon, Dr Nikos Evangelou and Dr Jonny Wilkinson for reviewing various drafts of this book, and Professor John Hampton and Dr David Gray for their support. We also wish to thank the doctors who taught us, and above all the patients who allowed us to examine them.

Abbreviations

ABG	Arterial blood gas	**DVLA**	Driver and Vehicle Licensing Agency
ACE	Angiotensin-converting enzyme	**DVT**	Deep vein thrombosis
ACTH	Adrenocorticotrophic hormone	**EBV**	Epstein–Barr virus
AF	Atrial fibrillation	**ECG**	Electrocardiogram
AFP	Alpha-fetoprotein	**EMG**	Electromyogram
AICD	Automated implantable cardiac defibrillator	**ESR**	Erythrocyte sedimentation rate
ANA	Anti-nuclear antibody	**FBC**	Full blood count
AR	Aortic regurgitation	**FEV$_1$**	Forced expiratory volume in 1 s
5-ASA	5-Aminosalicylic acid	**FTA**	Fluorescent treponema antibodies
ASD	Atrial septal defect	**FVC**	Forced vital capacity
AVR	Aortic valve replacement	**GH**	Growth hormone
BIPAP	Bilevel positive airway pressure	**Hb**	Haemoglobin
CABG	Coronary artery bypass graft	**HBV**	Hepatitis B virus
CAPD	Continuous ambulatory peritoneal dialysis	**HCG**	Human chorionic gonadotrophin
CCF	Congestive cardiac failure	**HCV**	Hepatitis C virus
CFA	Cryptogenic fibrosing alveolitis	**HGV**	Heavy goods vehicle
		HLA	Human lymphocyte antigen
CFTR	Cystic fibrosis transmembrane conductance regulator	**HOCM**	Hypertrophic obstructive cardiomyopathy
CK	Creatine kinase	**HRT**	Hormone replacement therapy
CML	Chronic myeloid leukaemia	**HSMN**	Hereditary sensory motor neuropathy
CMV	Cytomegalovirus	**HSV**	Herpes simplex virus
COPD	Chronic obstructive pulmonary disease	**IBD**	Inflammatory bowel disease
COMT	Catechol-o-methyl transferase	**IDDM**	Insulin-dependent diabetes mellitus
CRP	C-reactive protein	**IGF**	Insulin-like growth factor
CSF	Cerebrospinal fluid	**INR**	International normalized ratio
CVA	Cerebrovascular accident	**ITP**	Immune thrombocytopenic purpura
CXR	Chest X-ray (radiograph)		
DIPJ	Distal interphalangeal joint	**IV**	Intravenous
DM	Diabetes mellitus		

IVU	Intravenous urogram	**PUVA**	Psoralen ultraviolet A
JVP	Jugular venous pressure	**RA**	Rheumatoid arthritis
K_{CO}	Transfer coefficient	**RAD**	Right axis deviation
LAD	Left axis deviation	**RBBB**	Right bundle branch block
LDH	Lactate dehydrogenase	**RR**	Respiratory rate
LFT	Liver function test	**RV**	Right ventricle
LV	Left ventricle	**RVH**	Right ventricular
LVH	Left ventricular hypertrophy		hypertrophy
MAO	Monoamine oxidase	**Rx**	Treatment
MI	Myocardial infarction	**SCLC**	Small cell lung cancer
MND	Motor neurone disease	**SIADH**	Syndrome of inappropriate
MPTP	Methyl-phenyl-		anti-diuretic hormone
	tetrahydropyridine	**SLE**	Systemic lupus
MR	Mitral regurgitation		erythematosus
MRI	Magnetic resonance	**SOA**	Swelling of ankles
	imaging	**SSRI**	Selective serotonin reuptake
MCPJ	Metacarpophalangeal joint		inhibitor
MTPJ	Metatarsophalangeal joint	**SVCO**	Superior vena cava
MVR	Mitral valve replacement		obstruction
NIPPV	Non-invasive positive	T_4	Thyroxine
	pressure ventilation	*T* C	Temperature
NSAIDs	Non-steroidal	**TIA**	Transient ischaemic attack
	anti-inflammatory drugs	$T_L CO$	Carbon monoxide transfer
NSCLC	Non-small cell lung cancer		factor
OA	Osteoarthritis	**TOE**	Transoesophageal echo
Pa	Partial pressure	**TPHA**	*Treponema pallidum*
PBC	Primary biliary cirrhosis		haemagglutination assay
PEG	Percutaneous endoscopic	**TR**	Tricuspid regurgitation
	gastrostomy	**TSH**	Thyroid stimulating
PEFR	Peak expiratory flow rate		hormone
PIPJ	Proximal interphalangeal	**TTE**	Transthoracic echo
	joint	**U+E**	Urea and electrolytes
PRL	Prolactin	**UC**	Ulcerative colitis
PSV	Public service vehicle	**UTI**	Urinary tract infection
PTHrP	Parathyroid hormone related	**VSD**	Ventricular septal defect
	peptide	**WCC**	White cell count

Ethics, Law and Communication Skills

ETHICS AND LAW IN MEDICINE

Principles of medical ethics

Most ethical dilemmas can be resolved, at least in part, by considering the four cornerstones of any ethical argument, namely **autonomy, beneficence, non-maleficence and justice.**

Autonomy 'self-rule': respecting and following the patient's decisions in the management of their condition.

Beneficence: promoting what is in the patient's best interests.

Non-maleficence: avoiding harm.

Justice: doing what is good for the population as a whole. Distributing resources fairly.

There is often not a right or wrong answer to tricky ethical problems but this framework enables informed discussion:

Example:
• **PEG feeding a semi-conscious patient post-CVA.**

Autonomy: the patient wishes to be fed, or not.

Beneficence and **non-maleficence:** feeding may improve nutritional status and aid recovery, but with risks of complication from the insertion of the PEG tube and subsequent aspiration. Also the patient's poor quality of life may be lengthened.

Justice: heavy resource burden looking after PEG-fed patients in nursing homes.

In accepting a patient's autonomy to determine the course of management the clinician must be satisfied that the patient is competent. If this is not the case the doctor should act in the patient's best interests.

Competency and consent

Consent is only valid when the individual is competent (or in legal terms, 'has capacity').
• A patient is not incompetent because they act against their best interests.
• Capacity is not a global term but is specific to each decision, i.e. a patient may be competent to make a will but at the same time incompetent to consent to treatment.

- A clinician does not have to prove beyond all reasonable doubt that a patient has capacity, only that the balance of probability favours capacity.
- The three stages in assessing capacity are:
  1 Comprehension and retention of information needed to make the decision.
  2 Ability to believe the information, i.e. no delusion.
  3 Ability to weigh the information and make a decision.
- Patients under 16 yrs of age can consent to treatment if they are deemed 'Gillick competent', i.e. are deemed mature enough to understand the implications of their actions.

Legal aspects
A competent patient

> *Every human being of adult years and of sound mind has a right to determine what shall be done to his/her own body.*

- **Battery (assault):** a procedure or treatment that is performed without consent.
- **Negligence:** harm caused by a doctor acting outside accepted medical opinion or practice (Bolam Principle). If a patient does not receive certain relevant information when consented for a procedure a doctor may be found negligent. It is advisable to tell the patient of all potential serious complications and those with an incidence of at least 1%.

An incompetent patient

A doctor, by acting in the patient's best interests, can treat a patient against their will under common law.

- **Proxy consent:** a relative cannot consent on behalf of an incompetent patient.
- **Implied consent:** by going to hospital a patient should expect a nurse to take their blood pressure and therefore consent for this procedure need not necessarily be sought.
- **Advanced directives (living wills):** a patient makes a choice on their future medical care before they become incompetent. A doctor that treats a patient in the face of an advanced directive could be liable in battery.
- **Power of attorney:** a patient nominates a person (usually a relative) whilst competent to make decisions on their behalf if they were to become incompetent. However, this does not include medical management decisions.

- **Ward of court:** a doctor may apply to a judge to make medical decisions on behalf of the patient. This is advisable if it is not clear what the correct course of management should be and there is opposition from colleagues or relatives against the intended treatment.
- **The Mental Health Act 1983:** can only be evoked to treat psychiatric illness in non-consenting patients.

Section 5(2): emergency doctor's holding power
- Applied by one physician on an *in-patient* to enable a psychiatric assessment to be made.
- 72 h duration.
- Good practice to convert this to a Section 2.

Section 2: admission for assessment order
- Applied by two written medical recommendations (usually a psychiatrist and a GP) and an approved social worker or relative, on a patient *in the community*.
- 28 days duration.
- May be converted to a Section 3.
- The patient has a right of appeal to a tribunal within 14 days of detention.

Section 3: admission for treatment order
- Applied as in a Section 2 on a patient already diagnosed with a mental disorder.
- 3 months duration then reviewed.

Section 4: emergency admission to hospital order
- Applied by one doctor (usually a GP) and an approved social worker or relative.
- Urgent necessity is demonstrable.
- May be converted to a Section 2 or 3.

Confidentiality

GMC Guidance (*Confidentiality: Protecting and Providing Information,* September 2000, Section 1—Patients' right to confidentiality, Paragraph 1)

> *Patients have a right to expect that information about them will be held in confidence by their doctors. Confidentiality is central to trust between doctors and patients. Without assurances about confidentiality, patients may be reluctant to give doctors the information they need in order to provide good care.*

Legal aspects

- Under common law doctors are legally obliged to maintain confidentiality although this obligation is not absolute.
- Maintenance of confidentiality is a public not a private interest—it is in the public's interest to be able to trust a doctor. Therefore breaching confidentiality is a question of balancing public interests.
- Doctors have **discretion** to breach confidentiality when another party may be at serious risk of harm, e.g. an epileptic who continues to drive or an HIV-positive patient who refuses to tell their sexual partner. They may also share information within the medical team.
- Doctors **must** breach confidentiality to the relevant authorities in the following situations:
    - (i) Notifiable diseases
    - (ii) Drug addiction
    - (iii) Abortion
    - (iv) *In-vitro* fertilization
    - (v) Organ transplant
    - (vi) Births and deaths
    - (vii) Police request
    - (viii) Search warrant signed by a circuit judge
    - (ix) Court order
    - (x) Prevention, apprehension or prosecution of terrorists or perpetrators of serious crime.

The GMC provides guidelines on when confidentiality may be breached, which do not have the force of the law but are taken seriously by the courts. These guidelines may be consulted at: *www.gmc-uk.org*.

End of life decisions

This is a contentious area and medical opinion is diverse.

Killing vs. letting die
In the former, the doctor causes the patient's death, in the latter the patient's illness causes death, i.e. 'nature takes its course'. However, some disagree stating the doctor's inactivity causes death, which may make it more difficult to morally justify.

Withholding vs. withdrawing treatment
Although it may be emotionally easier to withhold treatment, rather than to withdraw that which has been started already, there are no legal or necessarily moral distinctions between the two.

Doctrine of double effect

This distinguishes actions that are intended to harm versus those where harm is foreseen but not intended. For example, administration of large doses of morphine to palliate a patient with a terminal illness may actually cause a respiratory arrest and subsequent death. It is morally acceptable though because the primary aim was to alleviate pain.

Do-not-resuscitate (DNR) orders

English law does not require doctors to prescribe futile treatments, even if requested to do so by the patient. Therefore a DNR order is an example of limiting treatment that is futile. Doctors should make a decision as to whether to inform the patient of this decision. It may be inhumane and distressing to raise issues of this nature with terminally ill patients.

Euthanasia

Euthanasia is intentional killing, i.e. murder under English law and therefore illegal. Assisted suicide, i.e. helping someone take their own life, is a criminal offence.

Arguments for

- Respecting a patient's autonomy over their body.
- Beneficence, i.e. 'mercy killing', may prevent suffering.
- Suicide is legal but is unavailable to the disabled.

Arguments against

- Good palliative care obviates the need for euthanasia.
- Risk of manipulation/coercion/exploitation of the vulnerable.
- Undesirable practices will occur when constraints on killing are loosened ('slippery-slope' argument).

COMMUNICATION SKILLS

Breaking bad news

If done well this can help the patient come to terms with their illness and minimize psychological distress. There are no hard and fast rules, but a patient-centred approach often helps.

How to do it
- Choose a setting that is private and free from disturbance (give your bleep to someone else). Have enough time to do it properly.
- Invite other health care workers, e.g. a nurse, for support and to ensure continuity of information given by all the team.
- Offer the opportunity for relatives to attend if the patient wishes. This is useful for patient support and can help the dissemination of information.
- Introduce yourself and the purpose of the discussion.
- Check the patient's existing awareness and gauge how much they want to be told.
- Give the bad news clearly and simply. Avoid medical jargon. Avoid information overload. Avoid 'loose terminology' that may be misinterpreted.
- Pause and acknowledge distress. Wait for the patient to guide the conversation and explore their concerns as they arise.
- Recap what has been discussed and check understanding.
- Bring the discussion to a close but offer an opportunity to speak again and elicit the help of other groups, e.g. specialist cancer nurses or societies, to help the patient at this difficult time.

Other problems
- **Denial**

If a patient is in denial reiterate the key message that needs to be addressed. Confront the inconsistencies in their perceptions and if this does not work, acknowledge their denial in a sensitive way. It may be better to leave this to a later date, perhaps when the patient is ready to confront the painful reality.

- **Anger**

This is a natural and usually transient part of the grieving process. 'Shooting the messenger' can occur occasionally, particularly if the news is delivered poorly. Acknowledge their anger and empathize

with their plight. If this does not diffuse the situation, terminate the session and reconvene later.
- **'How long have I got?'**
Answer in broad terms: hours–days, days–weeks, etc. Explore why the patient wants to know.

Dealing with a difficult patient

How to do it

An angry patient
- Listen without interruption and let them voice their anger.
- Keep calm and do not raise your voice.
- Acknowledge they are angry and try to explore why.
- Empathize.
- Apologize if there has been an error.
- If they feel they wish to take matters further then advise them of the trust's complaints procedure.

A non-compliant patient
- Explore why they have not taken their medication. Were the side effects bothering them? Was the drug not working?
- Educate the patient. Perhaps they were not aware how important it was to take the tablets.
- Offer solutions. Direct supervision of treatment, e.g. anti-tuberculosis treatment. Try alternative therapies.

A self-discharging patient
- Explain why you do not want them to leave.
- If they are competent they may leave but do so at their own risk and against medical advice. To stop them is assault.
- If they are incompetent, they can be detained by reasonable force, acting in their best interests under common law. To let them go is negligent. However, if in attempting to detain such a person there is risk of serious injury to the patient or those restraining the patient, then you may have no alternative but to let them go.

A patient that continues to drive despite contraindication
Although it is the duty of the patient (not the doctor) to declare a disability that precludes him/her from holding a UK driving licence, it is one of the acknowledged circumstances under which a breach of confidentiality may be justified.

- Try and persuade the patient to inform the DVLA. Mention lack of insurance cover if they drive and safety issues to themselves and other road users.
- Ask them to provide written evidence that they have informed the DVLA if you suspect they have not.
- Inform the patient that you will write to the DVLA if they fail to do so.
- Write to the DVLA if no evidence is forthcoming and to the patient to inform them you have done so.

Driving restrictions

Disease	Private vehicle licence	HGV/PSV licence
Epilepsy	**1 yr** Fit free **6 months** during treatment changes	**10 yrs** Fit free, off medication
MI	**1 month**	**3 months** Symptom free Completes 9 minutes of Bruce Protocol treadmill test
Stroke	**1 month**	**Banned** If persistent deficit
IDDM	**Notify DVLA**	**Banned**

Any illness where the doctor feels that the patient's ability to drive is significantly impaired should be referred to the DVLA for further action and the patient told not to drive in the mean time.

Other issues to address

- Explore the impact on the patient's job and lifestyle?
- How is the patient going to get home from your clinic?

For full guidelines: *www.dvla.gov.uk/at_a_glance/content.htm.*

Information delivery

Communication skills are frequently assessed by the candidate's ability to inform the patient about their medical condition.

How to do it

- Introduce yourself and establish the reason for the discussion.
- Assess the patient's level of knowledge.

- Give the information required in simple language avoiding medical jargon.
- Facilitate questions and answer them, but avoid digressing too much.
- Formulate a plan of action with the patient.
- Reiterate your discussion with the patient to ensure understanding.
- Offer further information sources, e.g. leaflets, societies or groups.
- Organize appropriate follow-up.
- Close the interview.

Tips

- Read the case scenario carefully and structure your interview in the 5 minutes beforehand.
- This is a role-play station so use your imagination.
- If you are asked a question by the patient and you do not know the answer, say that you are unable to answer at present but you will find out next time (as you would in real life!).
- Be aware of possible legal and ethical facets to the case and pre-empt the examiners by tackling them in the case before the discussion.
- Body language speaks volumes.

Worked examples

Epilepsy

An 18-year-old woman who is trying to become a professional model has had her second grand mal seizure in 3 months, which was witnessed by her GP. She has had a normal CT head and metabolic causes have been excluded. She has returned to your outpatient clinic for the results. Please discuss the diagnosis with her.

Points to discuss

- The diagnosis is epilepsy. Explain what this means to the patient in lay terms: *disorganized electrical activity in the brain.* **(See 'Information delivery' section.)**
- Explore **social aspects**:
  - She has been drinking a lot of alcohol recently and staying out late at all night parties.
  - She drives to modelling agencies and relies heavily on her car.
  - She hates taking tablets.
- Discuss **treatment** options to limit her seizure activity:
  - Avoid alcohol excess and sleep deprivation.
  - Avoid precipitants, e.g. flashing disco lights.

- Drugs: there are some newer anti-epileptic medications, e.g. Lamotrigine, that have fewer side-effects. This is important to her as she is a model!
- Stress **compliance (if poor compliance see 'Dealing with a difficult patient' section)**
  - It is imperative that if she is on the oral contraceptive combined pill, she is told the risks of **pill failure**. This is important, as anti-epileptics are teratogenic. Advise alternative forms of contraception, e.g. barrier or if this is unacceptable switch to a higher dose oestrogen pill or progesterone pill.
  - If she wants to become **pregnant,** it is a balance of risk between a seizure when pregnant, which carries a significant risk of miscarriage and the potential teratogenic side effects of the drugs. Most physicians encourage female patients wishing to start a family to continue on their epileptic treatment. Remember folate supplements!
- **Safety** issues
  - Avoid swimming or bathing alone and heights.
  - Driving restrictions **(if she continues to drive see 'Dealing with a difficult patient' and 'Breaking confidentiality' sections).**
- **Recap** the important points and formulate an agreed plan.
- **Check understanding** and answer her questions.
- **Other information:** offer leaflets, British Epilepsy Society (*www.epilepsy.org.uk*), contact numbers and an appointment with epilepsy specialist nurse.
- Conclude the interview.

Huntington's chorea

A 26-year-old son of your patient has requested to see you, to discuss his mother's diagnosis. She has developed a dementing illness and chorea in her late forties. Her father committed suicide at the age of 60. A diagnosis of Huntington's chorea has been made on genetic testing. She currently lives in her own home but is not coping. She has also asked her son to help her die. Discuss the relevant issues with her son. He is 'trying for a family'.

Points to discuss
- Ascertain that his mother has consented to this discussion to avoid the **confidentiality** pitfall, and a rather short interview!
  - **Remember if the mother is your patient and the son is not, you only have a duty of care to the mother. If she does not want you to discuss the diagnosis with her son, then to do so would breach confidentiality.**

- Explain Huntington's chorea and its inheritance to the son. **(See 'Information delivery' and 'Breaking bad news' sections.)** Emphasize that there is **no cure** and management is supportive.
- How the diagnosis **relates to him** and his family.
  - Anticipation, i.e. if he is affected the onset may be at an earlier age.
  - Genetic screening and family planning. Prenatal screening. This would involve abortion—briefly explore this with the patient.
  - Life insurance and employment implications.
- How the diagnosis **relates to his mother.**
  - Social aspects: community care or nursing home placement plans.
  - Legal aspects: advanced directives, power of attorney and ward of court may be discussed **(see 'Consent and competency' section).**
  - Assisted suicide is illegal **(see 'Death and dying' section).**
- **Recap** and formulate an agreed plan.
- **Check understanding** and answer questions.
- **Other information**: offer leaflets, Huntington's society contact numbers and an appointment with a geneticist. An appointment with a social worker would be useful to organize residential care for his mother.
- **Arrange follow-up** ideally with all the family as it affects all of them.
- Conclude the interview.

Paracetamol overdose

> *A patient arrives in the emergency medical unit having taken 50 Paracetamol tablets 4 h ago. She says she wants to die and does not want to be treated although she would like painkillers for her abdominal pain. Negotiate a treatment plan with this patient.*

Points to discuss

The overdose
- Be clear on the amount of Paracetamol taken and the time of ingestion as this will influence the management, i.e. calculating the treatment level of Paracetamol.
- Alcoholism or anti-epileptic medication lowers the treatment line.
- Assess the suicidal intent, e.g. letter.
- Previous psychiatric history.
- Negotiate an agreed **treatment plan** if possible.
- Organize a referral to the deliberate self-harm team.
- **Recap** and **check understanding.**
- Conclude the interview.

Treatment debate
- **Competency**
  - Does she understand that this overdose is life threatening and what the treatment involves?
  - Is the Paracetamol overdose affecting her judgement?
  - Is a psychiatric illness affecting her judgement, e.g. delusional?
- If deemed **incompetent** then you must act in her best interests and treat her against her will under **common law**.
- If **competent** she has a right to refuse treatment.

  If you do not treat and the patient dies, you may have to defend this decision in court. If you treat her in the face of her wishes, you could be charged with battery. Most courts will not find physicians that act in the patient's best interests guilty.

- **Implied consent**

  May be invoked to defend treatment of a patient that arrives in hospital having taken an overdose but they may have been taken there against their will, or they may have attended hospital to palliate their symptoms.

- **Advanced directives**

  Notes stating they do not wish to be treated should largely be ignored, because the attending physician cannot be sure of the circumstances in which it was written, e.g. under duress, or that the patient has not changed her mind.

- **The Mental Health Act** cannot be invoked to treat overdose patients, even if they have depression.
- Attempted suicide is no longer illegal in the UK. Assisting someone to commit suicide is illegal.

If in doubt it is prudent to treat overdose patients under common law, acting in their best interests.

Brain stem death and organ donation

You are working in intensive care and you have recently admitted a 30-year-old man who was hit by a car. He has sustained a severe head injury and his second assessment of brain stem tests show he is brain stem dead. You have found an organ donor card in his wallet. Please discuss the diagnosis with his mother and father and broach the subject of organ donation with them.

Points to discuss
Brain stem death
- Explain that he has had a severe brain injury and that he is brain dead (see 'Breaking bad news').

- **Inform them about brain death.**
- 'He has **died** and only the ventilator is keeping his other organs working.'
- Pause for reflection and questions.

Organ donation
- Broach in a sensitive way: 'I know this is a very difficult time for you both but did you know that your son carried a donor card?'
- Points that can be addressed may include:
  - The need for **an operation** to 'harvest' the organs.
  - **HIV testing** prior to donation.
  - Not all the organs taken may be used.
  - Time delays involved prior to the certification of death and the release of the body.
- Avoid information overload and be guided by the relative's questions and the time available.
- Offer to put them in touch with the **transplant coordinator** for the region. They will be able to counsel them further.
- Remind them that a decision has to be made swiftly but avoid harassing the relatives unduly (offer to come back when they have had a chance to think about it).

Being too involved in the transplantation program may be ethically wrong for an ITU physician, due to potentially conflicting interests.

A donor card is sufficient legal authority to proceed (advanced directive although the signature is not witnessed). However, it is good practice to assess the relatives' wishes and few centres would proceed if the relatives did not assent to organ donation.
- **Recap** and formulate a plan.
- **Check understanding** at each stage and answer their questions.
- **Offer other information**: leaflet on transplantation.
- Conclude the interview.

Discussion
- As in this case, discussion with a **coroner** must occur prior to organ donation if it is a coroner's case. Permission may be withheld if a death is due to a criminal action.
- **Human Tissue Act (1961) and Human Organ Transplant Act (1989)**
  - Guidelines and codes of practice on organ retrieval, consent and diagnostic tests of brain death.
- **Brain stem death**

Two consultants assess independently that:
- The cause of death is known and all potentially treatable causes for the patient's state have been excluded, e.g. hypothermia, biochemical derangement and drugs, i.e. the unconscious state is **irreversible** and **permanent.**
- The brain stem reflexes, e.g. pupil, corneal, motor cranial nerve responses, vestibulo-ocular, gag and cough reflexes are absent and there is no spontaneous respiratory drive at a $Paco_2 > 50\,mmHg$.
- **Organ donation**
  - All organs are usually harvested with minimum warm ischaemic time, i.e. with a beating heart up to the moment of harvesting (except corneas); hence these difficult discussions need to be addressed early.
  - Contraindications: infections, e.g. HIV and prion disease; metastatic tumours; severe atherosclerosis.
  - Be aware of the introduction of 'non-heart beating organ donation'.

For further information see GMC guidelines at *www.gmc-uk.org.*

Non-compliant diabetic

> *An 18-year-old female insulin-dependent diabetic has been admitted with yet another keto-acidotic episode. She has family problems. You notice she is very thin and has lanugo hair on her face. Please counsel her regarding her poor diabetic control and weight loss.*

Points to discuss
- **Diabetic education**
  - Review insulin regimen, injection sites and **compliance** (may be non-compliant due to weight gain or family problems).
  - Educate about the importance of tight glycaemic control and the dangers of diabetic ketoacidosis.
  - Ask about other cardiovascular risk factors, e.g. smoking.
- **Dieting and anorexia nervosa**
  - Emphasize the importance of a balanced diet and diabetic control.
  - Explore her dietary intake.
  - Ask her about her weight, body image and self-esteem.
  - Assess for **depression** (associated with anorexia).
- **Family problems**
  - Explore these and counsel. Patients suffering from anorexia often have problems at home.
  - **Family therapy** can be useful in treating anorexia nervosa.

- **Recap** and formulate a plan.
- **Check understanding** and answer questions.
- **Offer other information:** leaflets, Anorexia Nervosa Society.
- Conclude the interview.

Legal issues
- **Competency:** due to the effects of malnutrition on cognition, an anorexic patient may not be competent to refuse treatment.
- Anorexia nervosa can be treated under the **Mental Health Act (1983)** as an outpatient or in severe cases on a specialist unit.
- Food is deemed a treatment for a mental illness and can be given against the patient's will under the Mental Health Act.

Sample questions

Information delivery
- *This 60-year-old man is about to leave hospital, 7 days after an uncomplicated MI. He has some concerns regarding his return to normal life. What advice would you give him regarding his condition?*

- *A 23-year-old newly-diagnosed asthmatic has been recently discharged from hospital and arrives in your outpatient clinic for a review of his illness. He works as a veterinary nurse and smokes 15 cigarettes per day. Educate him about his illness, arrange further tests and instigate a treatment plan.*

- *A 36-year-old man has recently been diagnosed with acute myeloid leukaemia and has been sent to your clinic for assessment of his suitability for a bone marrow transplant. He has two siblings. Please discuss issues about his treatment with him.*

- *A 29-year-old man with a 14-year history of ulcerative colitis treated with steroids and ciclosporin has come to your follow-up clinic. He is concerned with some of the side-effects he has been having on his medication. Address this and counsel him in the further management of his condition.*

- *A 50-year-old heavy smoker presents with his fifth exacerbation of COPD this year. He tells you he does not take his inhalers because he thinks they make him worse. His blood gas on air reads a Pao_2 of 6.8. Discuss treatment options with him.*

Communicating medico-legal and ethical principles
- *A patient with longstanding multiple sclerosis is suffering from a flare of her disease. She has read on the Internet that there is a new treatment that might*

be helpful. Unfortunately, your trust has decided not to fund this treatment at present. Counsel her on these matters.

- *A patient's relatives arrive to be told that their father was unfortunately 'dead-on-arrival' to hospital. It is likely he suffered a large myocardial infarction. Break this bad news to them and guide them with regard to the need for a coroner's post-mortem. For religious reasons they would like the body released today.*

- *A 90-year-old woman who has recently had a debilitating stroke is classified as 'do not attempt resuscitation'. Her daughter has found out that this decision has been made without her consent and demands that her mother be for resuscitation. Discuss the management of this patient with the daughter.*

- *A patient with motor neurone disease who is now wheelchair-bound has come to your clinic. She believes she is a burden to her family and wants your advice regarding the best way to end her own life. Please counsel her.*

- *A 24-year-old doctor has come to your clinic. She has recently been on elective to Africa where she sustained a needle stick injury. Initial tests show she is hepatitis C positive. She is reluctant to stop working. Please counsel her.*

History Taking

Introduction and advice

Prior to entering the room you will have 5 minutes to read the 'GP referral letter'. Then you will take a history from the patient in front of both examiners. At the end of 14 minutes the patient will leave the room and you will have a minute to gather your thoughts before 5 minutes of discussion with the examiners. You should not present the history back to them, but rather produce a problem list to discuss.

The format of this section will teach you how to do this.

Surprisingly more candidates fail this station than any other. Yet it is often ignored in exam preparation.

There are essentially two types of history you will encounter. In one the patient presents with a collection of symptoms and you must attempt to reach a diagnosis. In the other the patient has a chronic disease where the diagnosis is clear but you must review previous investigation, treatments and search out possible complications. Examples of both of these will be presented.

Take note of the following points. **Many of these are specifically mentioned on the examiner's mark sheet.**

- **Use preparation time wisely**
Before you enter the room you will have 5 minutes to read the GP letter. You will be provided with blank paper, which you may take into the room. Use this time to note down a written structure for the interview with key points that you must not forget when the adrenaline is flowing! For example, in a diagnosis question a written list of differentials will prompt you to ask appropriate questions to support or refute each. This helps you reach the final diagnosis in a logical and systematic way and scores more marks than an apparently jumbled sequence of questions.

- **Take a complete history**
Systems Review, Past Medical History, Family History, Drug History, Smoking and Alcohol are all specifically mentioned on the mark sheet. You will lose points for neglecting them. Actors may be primed to give you certain information only if specifically questioned upon it.

- **Explore psychosocial issues**
The impact the condition has on his or her relationships, family and job is crucial and in the exam, patients will probably not volunteer this unless asked. In most cases this should feature on your subsequent list of problems.

• **Attempt to develop a rapport**

The way you interact with the patient is assessed. Attempt to put them at ease. Respond appropriately to things they tell you—do not say 'good' after hearing about their recent bereavement! Appear sympathetic if required. Maintain appropriate levels of eye contact. Balance open and closed questions.

• **Review information with patient**

Again this is specifically mentioned on the mark sheet but is often neglected. Tell the patient you would like to check you have the story straight. Not only does this confirm the facts but may well clarify things to you that had not been apparent before.

• **Adhere to a time structure**

There will be a clock in the room that will be easily visible to you. You have 14 minutes with the patient. You will throw away marks if you do not finish within time. Clearly each case will vary but as a rough guide aim to spend 5 minutes on the presenting complaint, 4 minutes on past medical, drug and family histories, and 4 minutes on social history. This leaves you 1 minute to review information with the patient and then a further minute to get your thoughts straight for the discussion.

• **Generate a problem list**

By now you should have generated a list of the main issues pertinent to the case. This may be a single diagnosis but may be an extensive list including medical problems, social problems and concerns or complaints about treatment. This will form the crux of your discussion.

• **Think ahead about your discussion**

This is likely to involve questions on further investigation and management, so anticipate this as you go along.

Scoring well on this station requires good exam technique. It is rather different to the history you take daily at work and it is also the station that most candidates underestimate during preparation for the exam.

What follows are 10 typical examples that we suggest you practise in small groups. The cases are introduced with a GP letter. We also include a briefing to be read only by the person role-playing the patient. At the end there is a suggested problem list to compare with your own along with likely discussion points. You must practise these with strict timings and ideally with others observing. You must be used to taking a complete and logical history and having your problem list ready for discussion at the 15-minute point.

As in the exam the cases are deliberately varied. Some focus on a single medical problem while others involve multiple medical and social issues. The cases are based on real PACES cases.

Case 1

Dear Dr,

I would be grateful if you could see this 50-year-old lady who is new to my practice and has had rheumatoid arthritis for 5 yrs. Her symptoms are currently not well controlled on Arthrotec® and Coprox-amol.

Case 2

Dear Dr,

I would be grateful for your assessment of this 55-year-old man with poorly controlled diabetes. He has previously been reluctant to attend a diabetic clinic. He is currently taking oral hypoglycaemic medication and Bendrofluazide. I feel he may need to start insulin soon. I calculated his body mass index today at 36. His last HbA_{1c} was 11.4.

Case 3

Dear Dr,

This 26-year-old female attended my surgery today complaining of difficulty walking that had come on over a few days. On examination she has a markedly ataxic gait but no other abnormality. She has no significant past medical history and takes only simple analgesia for headaches. I would be grateful for your urgent assessment.

Case 4

Dear Dr,

Thank you for seeing this 35-year-old teacher urgently. I am concerned she has had a pulmonary embolus. She developed central pleuritic chest pain during the course of yesterday; however, she has felt generally unwell for a week. She was on the combined oral contraceptive pill until 1 yr ago. She currently takes Fluoxetine for depression and Nifedipine for Raynaud's syndrome.

On examination she was a little breathless. Pulse 100 BP 170/100. Chest clear.

Case 5

Dear Dr,

I would be grateful if you would see this 22-year-old language student who has had persistent diarrhoea since returning from Russia 2 months ago. Several of her friends on her trip also had diarrhoea whilst abroad but unlike them her symptoms have not settled with antibiotics.

Case 6

Dear Dr,

I would be grateful for your opinion on this 78-year-old man who has recurrent dizzy spells and on two occasions he has blacked out at home. He had a pacemaker inserted 2 yrs ago following an episode of heart block, which complicated an anterior myocardial infarction. I wondered if the pacemaker was malfunctioning, though a recent check was satisfactory. His only other medical history is hypertension. In the surgery today his pulse was 70 regular and BP 135/85.

Case 7

Dear Dr,

Thank you for seeing this 56-year-old man because his wife has noticed he is yellow. Apart from looking a bit jaundiced there was no abnormality on physical examination today. His liver function tests are chronically deranged. An ultrasound of his abdomen was reported as normal. He has a history of ulcerative colitis for which he had a colectomy in 1990. Otherwise he is well and only takes Bendrofluazide for hypertension.

Case 8

Dear Dr,

Thank you for seeing this 30-year-old shop assistant who complains of amenorrhoea for 6 months. She has a history of manic depression for which she is under psychiatric review but is currently well and off medication. A pregnancy test was negative. Her body mass index was calculated at 25.

Case 9

Dear Dr,

We have had this 30-year-old man on our asthma clinic registry since he was a teenager although he has never been very diligent about attending his appointments. However, he now complains that his breathing has been getting very much worse over the last few months and his symptoms are not controlled with Ventolin and Becotide. I would be grateful for your opinion.

Case 10

Dear Dr,

Many thanks for seeing this 20-year-old man who feels increasingly fatigued and unwell. On examination he has bilateral cervical lymphadenopathy, which has been increasing for at least 2 months. There are no nodes elsewhere and there is no other abnormality on physical examination.

Case 1

Briefing for patient

You are 50 years old.

About 5 yrs ago you first noticed both hands and wrists were intermittently painful and swollen especially in the morning. If asked, these joints were often quite stiff for several hours after getting up each morning. Symptoms eased a little as the day went on.

Since then your feet and left hip have also started to become painful.

Your previous GP had diagnosed rheumatoid arthritis 4 yrs ago on the basis of X-rays of the hands and a blood test. You have been taking Coproxamol, Arthrotec® and Prednisolone since then. The dose of Prednisolone has varied between 5 mg and 20 mg depending on symptom severity. He had talked about referring you to a specialist in the past but as the tablets seemed to control symptoms reasonably well you did not really see the need to consult another doctor.

Recently, however, the pain and stiffness is worse making it difficult to manage with housework. You have particular difficulty holding heavy saucepans and opening jars, and your husband now has to do much of the cooking. The swelling is starting to make your hands look a little funny. Walking is uncomfortable on the balls of your feet unless you wear padded shoes such as trainers. Your hip rarely causes much trouble.

Commonly you wake up at night with a burning pain in both hands. This seems mainly to affect the thumbs, index and middle fingers. It eventually goes away with shaking your hands.

Six years ago you had a hysterectomy for heavy periods.
You have never had problems with your liver or lungs. You are not breathless. You have never broken a bone.
You are otherwise fit and well.
Your only tablets are Coproxamol, Arthrotec and Prednisolone 5 mg daily. You are not aware of the need for 'bone protection' when on long-term steroids.

You worked as a secretary until you had your two children 10 yrs ago. Since then you have been a housewife. You are happily married and your husband is a solicitor.
Your parents are both fit and well as are your children and brother.
You have never smoked and drink an occasional glass of wine.

Problem list

- Increasingly symptomatic rheumatoid disease interfering significantly with daily life. This is despite treatment with NSAIDs.
- Not previously used **disease-modifying agents** such as Methotrexate. From the history there is no obvious contraindication.
- Excessive use/requirement for corticosteroids resulting in **significant risks of osteoporosis** especially with hysterectomy at a relatively early age. Disease modifying drugs should allow a gradual reduction of steroid dose. Appropriate to consider bone protection, e.g. HRT or alendronate.
- Symptoms suggestive of **bilateral carpal tunnel syndrome**.
- No other complications of rheumatoid suggested by the history, e.g. pulmonary or pleural involvement or anaemia.

Discussion

- Systemic complications of rheumatoid arthritis.
- Treatment of rheumatoid disease and the use of disease modifying drugs such as Methotrexate and Infliximab and symptomatic relievers like the Cox-2 inhibitors.
- Osteoporosis and bone protection.

Case 2

Briefing for patient

You are 55 years old.

Diabetes was diagnosed 10 yrs ago and initially treated with diet alone. When this was not successful, tablets were introduced by your GP and the doses gradually increased.
You currently take Metformin 850 mg t.d.s., Gliclazide 160 mg b.d. and Bendrofluazide 2.5 mg daily. You generally take your tablets as prescribed because your wife nags you to.

Your eyesight is good and you have regular checks at an ophthalmologist.
You are aware of the importance of looking after your feet and have no foot ulcers.
Other than high blood pressure you have no other medical problems. Your cholesterol has never been checked.

You work as an HGV driver.
You smoke 30 cigarettes a day.
You drink very little alcohol.
You are aware your diet is not good and that you are rather overweight.
You take very little exercise.

You are happily married with two children aged 5 and 8.
Diabetes runs in your family—father and both brothers.
Your father had a heart attack at the age of 55 and your brother recently had a bypass operation. This worries you although you have had no heart problems to your knowledge.

Problem list

- **Poorly controlled diabetes** on maximal oral hypoglycaemic treatment.
- **Obesity** will exacerbate insulin resistance and is likely to be made worse by starting insulin. Weight loss will improve glycaemic control as well as reducing cardiovascular risk.
- **High risk for ischaemic heart disease**. Smoking must be addressed. Check lipids and if necessary treat. Hypertension should be aggressively controlled ideally with an ACE inhibitor, e.g. Ramipril, which has additional cardio-protection properties.
- Starting insulin would result in **loss of HGV license**.

Discussion

- Management: he is likely to need insulin but this will result in the loss of his job. A serious attempt to lose weight should first be made. This may improve glycaemic control sufficiently to delay the need for insulin. Reduction of cardiac risk is a major component of his management.
- Complications of diabetes, e.g. retinopathy, neuropathy, nephropathy and atherosclerosis, their identification and management.
- Evidence to support the use of ACE inhibitors in diabetes, e.g. HOPE trial.

Case 3

Briefing for patient

You are a 26-year-old student who is normally fit and well.

For the last week you have had difficulty walking and keep stumbling over to the right. As a result you have been unable to play hockey this week. Your friends say you look as if you are drunk. The severity varies a little from day to day but was most severe two nights ago. If specifically asked, this followed a long soak in the bath.

Your speech is normal and your arms seem OK. You have not had a fit or a blackout. You get headaches when you are tired or stressed. The headaches are eased with Paracetamol. The headaches have perhaps been a little worse recently. They come on late in the day and have never occurred in the morning on waking. They are not associated with nausea.

This time last year your speech went funny for a few days while on holiday, but it resolved before you saw a doctor. It is difficult to describe it but it sounded funny and slightly slurred.

If specifically asked, you may volunteer the fact that your vision became quite blurred in your right eye for about a week several months ago. The eye also felt painful at the time. Then it came back to normal. Around the same time you had a few episodes when you wet yourself in bed. You were very embarrassed about this but it has not recurred.

You have no other medical problems.
You take no medications at all.
You drink five pints of beer at weekends but not during the week.
You do not smoke.
Both parents are fit and well. You are an only child.

Problem list

- **Truncal ataxia** with a background of symptoms suggesting **optic neuritis,** dysarthria and urinary incontinence. The **relapsing/remitting** nature of these symptoms, separated in time and location, in a young adult is virtually diagnostic of **Multiple Sclerosis**. This is supported further by the presence of Uthoff's phenomenon (worsening of symptoms by heat—in this case a hot bath).
- The headaches sound like simple **tension headaches** and do not require further investigation.

Discussion

- Investigation and management of multiple sclerosis.
- Differential diagnosis of headaches.
- Socio-economic impact of chronic disability.

Case 4

Briefing for patient
You are a 35-year-old teacher.

You have felt generally unwell and run down for several months.
You have felt hot and shivery for a few weeks. Yesterday you noticed pain in the centre of your chest. The pain is sharp and grating. It hurts when you breathe in deeply. The only position you are comfortable in is sitting upright and last night you could not sleep lying down because of the pain. Exertion and eating do not affect the pain.

You are not short of breath. Your legs do not swell up; you have not been on an airline recently, and have not been immobilized either.

For years you have had Raynaud's Syndrome treated with Nifedipine by the GP. Your hands get very cold and turn white, blue and then red if you do not wear gloves in winter. Recently your wrists and hand joints are intermittently painful to the point that it is sometimes hard to write at work.

Two years ago you were admitted with sharp pains in left side of chest and suspicion of a clot on the lung. However, the VQ scan was normal and you were discharged.

If asked, you have no skin rash currently; however, you react badly to the sun and easily get burned especially across your face.

You have felt very depressed recently and have been off work intermittently for 3 months. You feel too run down to work at the moment. Antidepressants are not really working. You work as a relief teacher and are not paid if you do not work. The lack of income is a major problem at home as your husband has recently been made redundant.

You do not smoke but admit to drinking too much—roughly a bottle of wine per day.

Your parents are both alive and well, and you do not have any siblings. You have one healthy 4-year-old boy (you had three miscarriages in your 20s).

Problem list
- The presenting problem is suggestive of **acute pericarditis**.
- She also describes a background of non-specific ill health with **Raynaud's** phenomenon, **polyarthritis**, **photosensitivity** and previous **pleurisy**.

- This collection of symptoms suggests an underlying connective tissue disease such as **SLE**.
- Remember also the **hypertension** noted by the GP. Possible renal involvement.
- She feels **depressed**, perhaps due to the symptoms of her disease or perhaps caused directly by SLE.
- The disease is causing significant **work, family** and **financial problems**.
- Her **alcohol** intake is above the recommended safe levels.

Discussion
- Management of acute pericarditis.
- Complications of SLE.
- Further investigation and management of SLE.
- Given her miscarriages anti-phospholipid syndrome might be discussed.

Case 5

Briefing for patient

You are a 22-year-old university language student who returned 2 months ago from a year in Russia as part of your course. Your final exams are in 3 months time.

About 3 months ago while in Russia, you developed diarrhoea. This has continued since then although not as bad. In Russia, the diarrhoea was occurring up to 10 times a day; now it occurs around three times a day. You usually have little warning and are occasionally incontinent. You are very embarrassed about talking about this.

On direct questioning, there is red blood mixed in with the diarrhoea normally preceded by cramping lower abdominal pains. Often you have the sensation of needing to go but are unable to produce anything when you try to open your bowels.

You have not lost weight nor had any fevers. You ate Russian food for the whole year and it had not previously upset you. A couple of your friends developed diarrhoea. They were told it was Giardiasis and they got better with antibiotics. Your GP has tried this but it has not really helped.

In the past you have been fit and active although troubled a little recently by lower back pain. This started about a year ago. It is worse in the mornings and usually eases within a few hours of getting up. Sometimes you take Ibuprofen when it is bad. No other joints are painful. In Russia you also developed unexplained painful bruising on your shins, which gradually went away after a few weeks. You thought nothing of it and would not mention this unless asked about skin rashes.

You do not smoke. You drink in moderation. You live in a hall of residence and are currently studying for your exams. The only medicine you ever take is Ibuprofen for backache. Your mother, father and sister are all fit and healthy.

Problem list

- Persistent bloody diarrhoea and tenesmus is suggestive of **ulcerative colitis**.
- A history compatible with both **sacroiliitis** and **erythema nodosum** is evident and associated with ulcerative colitis.

- Giardiasis, whilst common in Eastern Europe and Russia, does not cause bloody diarrhoea. Other infectious causes of bloody diarrhoea, e.g. *Shigella* and *Salmonella*, should be excluded by stool microscopy and culture.
- There is anxiety about incontinence during her imminent exams.

Discussion
- Differential diagnosis and investigation of bloody diarrhoea.
- Management of colitis.

Case 6

Briefing for patient
You are 78 years old.

Over the last 2 months you have suffered from recurrent dizzy spells. Sometimes these are bad enough that you have to sit or lie down for a few minutes before it resolves. The room does not actually spin around but you feel very light-headed and faint. Last week you actually collapsed in your bedroom after getting up to pass water in the night. You did not hurt yourself nor did you wet yourself and once you took it steady you were able to get to the toilet. You were not out for long and knew exactly what had happened afterwards. A similar thing has happened before while you were washing up. As it starts, you sometimes get tunnel vision and feel sweaty before you collapse.

You have no chest pain, palpitations or breathlessness either at rest or on exertion. The attacks are not related to moving your head around and you have no ear problems. There have been no problems with your speech or limbs. These attacks have never occurred while sitting or lying down. If you stand up too quickly the symptoms occur.

In the past you have had a heart attack and needed a pacemaker afterwards. This was checked 3 weeks ago and was said to be fine. The blackouts you had then were different, occurring without warning whilst sitting or standing. You have mild heart failure but this has been well controlled lately and you are able to walk to the shops easily. You have had high blood pressure in the past but recently this has been lower according to your GP. Your Ramipril dose was increased at a hospital appointment about 3 months ago.

You live alone. You normally cope fine, but are currently very worried about what would happen if you had a fall and hurt yourself as there is no one nearby that you could phone. You do not smoke or drink.

Problem list
- The story is suggestive of **postural hypotension** and the ACE inhibitor is the likely culprit.
- Excluded other causes of dizziness and collapse:
  - **Cardiac:** arrhythmia/aortic stenosis.
  - **Neurological:** posterior circulation TIAs/epilepsy.
  - **Other:** micturation syncope, carotid sinus sensitivity, vasovagal.

- The patient lives alone and falls jeopardize his independence. Perhaps a 'lifeline' alarm system would be appropriate.

Discussion
- Falls and syncope in the elderly.
- Side-effects of ACE inhibitors.

Case 7

Briefing for patient
You are 56 years old.

Recently your wife has commented you look jaundiced which is why you went to the doctor. Looking back you have been a little tired recently and have lost about 9 lb in weight. Your skin has been intermittently very itchy and you have been scratching a lot. You have had some very minor vague aches in the right side of your abdomen but nothing severe. You have not had a fever. There have been no other symptoms.

You have travelled abroad only to France recently. You have never been outside Europe. You have not been in contact with anyone jaundiced.
You have never used IV drugs although did smoke cannabis as a student. You have no tattoos.
You drink two or three pints of beer at weekends but have never drunk heavily.
You do not smoke.
You are happily married with two children. Apart from your wife you have had no other sexual partners.
You work as a salesman and have no exposure to sewage, drains or outdoor water.

You had ulcerative colitis diagnosed as a teenager and finally had a colectomy in 1990. The operation was complicated by a post-op bleed for which you needed to return to theatre. You were given a large blood transfusion. You have had no problems from your UC recently.

Your GP started you on Bendrofluazide 2 yrs ago for hypertension. You take no other over-the-counter or herbal medication.

Both your parents and your brother are fit and healthy.

Problem list
- In the presence of longstanding ulcerative colitis, abnormal liver function tests with a normal ultrasound and nothing in the history to suggest an alternative cause raises the possibility of **Primary Sclerosing Cholangitis**.
- It is important to explore other causes of abnormal liver function tests, in particular alcohol, medications and risks for chronic viral hepatitis.
- The blood transfusion was in 1990 and therefore should be clear of the hepatitis C virus.

Discussion

- Investigation of a jaundiced patient.
- Investigation and treatment of primary sclerosing cholangitis.

Case 8

Briefing for patient

You are a 30-year-old shop assistant.

Over the last year your periods have become progressively more irregular and you have now not had a period at all for 6 months. Otherwise you feel well. You do not think you could be pregnant as you have used barrier contraception with your current partner and two pregnancy tests have been negative.

You exercise normally but not excessively and eat a normal diet.
You have no symptoms of hot or cold intolerance and do not suffer with palpitations or tremor and your bowels are normal. You do not suffer from dizziness or faints or excessive thirst.
You do not suffer with indigestion.
You do not have headaches.
You do not have a problem with your vision, but recently crashed your car because 'a car came out of no-where'.
You have noticed that you have been lactating over the past few weeks. You are embarrassed but also quite worried about this and would only divulge this personal information if asked in a direct but sensitive way.

You had an operation on your neck 3 yrs ago for high calcium levels, which was diagnosed after you had a small kidney stone.

You saw a psychiatrist around the same time for depression and take Prozac intermittently when you feel like it. You have taken no other medication.

Your mother and sister are fit and well. Your father died in his 50s from a bleeding ulcer for which he had previously had surgery. You think he also had an operation on his neck at some stage.

You do not smoke and rarely drink alcohol.

You are happily married and keen to start a family in the near future.

Problem list
- Amenorrhoea and galactorrhoea are suggestive of a pituitary adenoma including a **prolactinoma.**
- **Dopamine antagonists,** e.g. anti-psychotics, can cause hyperprolactinaemia but rarely SSRIs, and in this case their prescription preceded the symptoms by 2 yrs.

- **Other pituitary** function appears to be normal.
- Crashing the car may have been due to **bi-temporal hemianopia.**
- The background of **hyperparathyroidism** ('bones, **stones,** abdominal groans and **psychic moans'**) and the **family history** suggestive of hyperparathyroidism and recurrent peptic ulceration (gastrinoma) suggests **Multiple Endocrine Neoplasia type I (MEN I).**
- She wants to have children but is currently likely to be **infertile.**

Discussion
- Investigation of a pituitary adenoma and management.
- Details of MEN I.
- Causes of secondary amenorrhoea. Referral to a fertility specialist and genetic counselling may be needed once the pituitary lesion has been treated.

Case 9

Briefing for patient
You are 30 years old and were first diagnosed with asthma as a teenager.

Until recently your symptoms have never been very severe and consisted of cough at night and intermittent wheezy days. Ventolin® has always been very effective. You did not go to your GP asthma clinic because your breathing was never very bad and all they did was nag you about smoking. You have never been admitted to hospital with asthma.

Over the last few months, however, your breathing has been getting steadily worse. Your asthma is particularly bad in the evenings with cough, wheezing and breathlessness, which prevent you from going out when severe. Now your breathing is bad most nights. You have not coughed up any sputum and have not had a fever. You have had no pain in your chest.

There have been days when your chest is fine and on a recent family holiday to France you had no symptoms at all and your exercise tolerance was unlimited.

There is nothing at home that seems to precipitate the asthma. You have no pets or birds. Your sister has a cat that has always made your asthma worse when you visit her house but you have not been there recently.

You work in a car factory on a production line. You are not involved in the spray painting although it does happen nearby. You do not wear a mask. The spray sometimes causes a runny nose and cough but does not seem to cause the wheezing as this only comes on later in the afternoons and evening. However, your symptoms do seem to be a bit better at weekends and were much better when away on holiday for a week.

You have been doing this job for a year now and enjoy working and earning good money. Previously you were unemployed for nearly 2 yrs and you had to go on the dole to support your wife and two small children. You almost got a divorce during this time and you blame 'money problems' for almost wrecking your marriage.

You are currently using a Salbutamol inhaler. You have a Becotide inhaler but rarely use this as it makes very little difference.

You smoke five cigarettes per day and are trying to cut down. You do not drink alcohol.

Your parents and brother are fit and have no respiratory problems

Problem list

- A deterioration in asthma with a temporal relationship to work suggests **occupational asthma**. It is not uncommon for onset of symptoms to be delayed for a few hours after exposure. The history of relief of symptoms during holiday is typical. Spray painting is one of the commonest causes of occupational asthma.
- **Poor compliance and asthma education** are also playing a role.
- Continued smoking is a problem.
- **Financial problems** and difficulty finding work are relevant.

Discussion

- Might involve further investigation of asthma by peak-flow diaries to confirm the relationship between work and asthma.
- Occupational asthma management may also be covered (the only effective treatment is avoidance of precipitant).
- Employees with occupational asthma are eligible for industrial injury benefit.

Case 10

Briefing for patient
You are a 20-year-old English student.

For the last 4 months you have been troubled by recurrent coughs and colds. You have intermittently coughed up yellow sputum but no blood. You now feel you have no energy and are completely unable to study. You noticed some lumps in your neck recently, which have been enlarging.

If asked:
You have not had a sore throat or a rash.
You have not travelled abroad other than to Spain 2 yrs ago.
You have no contact with TB.
You have no pets.
You have lost about 14 lb in weight over the last 2 months.
You have had to change bedclothes almost daily due to drenching night sweats.

You have not used IV drugs.
You are homosexual and have had one partner for a year. Neither of you have had an HIV test.
You used to drink a lot of alcohol but have recently found that you feel awful when you drink and your neck hurts a lot so you have abstained totally for the last month.
You smoke 20 cigarettes per day.
You have never been ill before nor taken any medication.
Your family members are all fit and well.

Problem list
- Lymphadenopathy, weight loss and drenching night sweats are suggestive of lymphoma, in particular **Hodgkin's disease.**
- Other differentials include
  - Infection: **HIV, glandular fever, TB.**
  - Inflammatory: sarcoid, connective tissue disease.
  - Solid tumour: **adenocarcinoma**, melanoma (smokes but young age).
  - Drugs

Discussion
- Differential diagnosis.
- Investigations of lymphadenopathy and diagnosis of Hodgkin's disease: Reed–Sternberg cells on lymph node biopsy.
- Management issues.

Cardiology and Neurology

Aortic stenosis

This patient presents with increasing dyspnoea. Examine his cardiovascular system to elucidate the cause.

Clinical signs

- Slow rising, low volume pulse.
- Narrow pulse pressure.
- Apex beat is sustained in stenosis (**HP**: **h**eaving **p**ressure-loaded).
- Thrill in aortic area (right sternal edge, 2nd intercostal space).
- Auscultation:

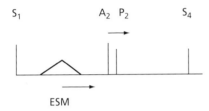

An ejection systolic murmur (ESM) loudest in the aortic area and radiating to the carotids.

Severity:
soft and delayed A$_2$
delayed (not loud) ESM
S$_4$

Extra points

Complications

- **Endocarditis:** splinters, Osler's nodes (finger pulp), Janeway lesions (palms), Roth spots (retina), temperature, splenomegaly and haematuria.
- **Left ventricular dysfunction:** dyspnoea, displaced apex, bibasal crackles.
- **Conduction problems: acute,** endocarditis; **chronic,** calcified aortic valve node.

Differential diagnosis

- HOCM.
- VSD.
- Aortic sclerosis: normal pulse character and no radiation of murmur.
- Aortic flow.

Discussion

Causes: ABCS

- **A**ge (senile degeneration and calcification).
- **B**icuspid.

- Congenital (valvular, supravalvular, subaortic membrane).
- Streptococcal associated (rheumatic fever and rarely bacterial endocarditis).

Associations
- Coarctation and bicuspid aortic valve.
- Angiodysplasia.

Severity
- **Symptoms**   **50% mortality @**
  Chest pain   5 yrs
  Dyspnoea   2 yrs
  Syncope   18 months
- **Signs**
  Auscultation features.
  Left ventricular failure.
  Right ventricular failure is preterminal.
- **Investigations**
  - **ECG:** LVH on voltage criteria, conduction defect.
  - **CXR:** often normal; calcified valve.
  - **Echo:** gradient >50 mmHg (>100 mmHg severe).
  - **Catheter:** aortic gradient and coronary angiography (coronary artery disease often coexists with aortic stenosis).

Treatment
- **Asymptomatic**
  - None.
  - Regular review 6/12.
  - Antibiotic prophylaxis for dental, genitourinary and colonic investigations or treatments.
- **Symptomatic**
  - Aortic valve replacement +/− CABG.
  - Operative mortality 2–5%.
  - Ideally operate just before LV dysfunction occurs.

Duke's Criteria for infective endocarditis
Major:
- Typical organism in two blood cultures.
- Echo: abscess, vegetation, dehiscence.

Minor:
- Pyrexia >38°C.
- Echo suggestive.

- Predisposed, e.g. prosthetic valve.
- Embolic phenomena.
- Vasculitic phenomena (ESR↑, CRP↑).
- Atypical organism on blood culture.

Diagnose if the patient has 2 major, 1 major and 2 minor, or 5 minor criteria.

Aortic incompetence

This patient has been referred by his GP with 'a new murmur'. He is asymptomatic. Please examine his cardiovascular system and diagnose his problem.

Clinical signs
- Collapsing pulse.
- Wide pulse pressure, e.g. 180/45.
- Apex beat is hyperkinetic and displaced laterally (**TV**: thrusting volume-loaded).
- Thrill in the aortic area.
- Auscultation.

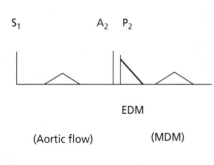

Early diastolic murmur (EDM) loudest at the lower left sternal edge with the patient sat forward in expiration.

There may be an aortic flow murmur and a mid-diastolic mumur (MDM) (Austin–Flint).

In severe AR the EDM and systolic flow murmur are loud and obliterate the second heart sound.

Extra points
- **Severity:** collapsing pulse, wide pulse pressure, pulmonary oedema.
- **Cause:** endocarditis; connective tissue disease, e.g. Marfan's, ankylosing spondylitis; syphilis (Argyll Robertson pupil).
- **Eponymous signs**
  - Corrigan's: visible vigorous neck pulsation.
  - Quincke's: nail bed capillary pulsation.
  - De Musset's: head nodding.
  - Duroziez's: diastolic murmur proximal to femoral artery compression.
  - Traube's: 'pistol shot' sound over the femoral arteries.

Discussion
Causes
- Congenital, e.g. membranous VSD.

- Acquired:

	Acute	Chronic
Valve leaflet	Endocarditis	Rheumatic fever
		Connective tissue disease, e.g. RA
Aortic root	Dissection (type A)	Dilatation: Marfan's, hypertension
	Trauma	Aortitis: syphilis, ankylosing spondylitis

Other causes of a collapsing pulse
- Pregnancy
- Patent ductus arteriosus
- Paget's disease
- Anaemia
- Thyrotoxicosis

Investigation
- **ECG:** lateral T-wave inversion.
- **CXR:** cardiomegaly, widened mediastinum and pulmonary oedema.
- **TTE/TOE:**
  Severity: LV function and dimensions, root dimensions.
  Cause: intimal dissection flap or vegetation.
- **Cardiac catheterization:** grade severity and check coronary patency.

Management
Surgery
Acute:
- Dissection.
- Aortic root abscess/endocarditis (homograft preferably).

Chronic
Replace the aortic valve when:
- **Symptomatic:** dyspnoea and reduced exercise tolerance.
OR
- **The following criteria are met:**
  1 pulse pressure >100 mmHg.
  2 ECG changes.
  3 LV enlargement on CXR.
Ideally replace the valve prior to significant left ventricular dilatation and dysfunction.

Prognosis
There is 65% mortality at 3 yrs if the above three criteria are present.

Mitral stenosis

This patient has been complaining of reduced exercise tolerance.
Examine his heart and elucidate the cause of his symptoms.

Clinical signs

- Malar flush.
- Irregular pulse if AF is present.
- Tapping apex (palpable 1st heart sound).
- Left parasternal heave if pulmonary hypertension is present or enlarged left atrium.
- Auscultation:

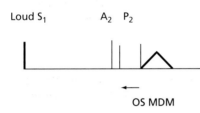

Loud S_1 A_2 P_2

OS MDM

Loud 1st heart sound. Opening snap (OS) of mobile mitral leaflets opening followed by a mid-diastolic murmur (MDM), which is best heard at the apex, in the left lateral position in expiration with the bell. Presystolic accentuation of the MDM occurs if the patient is in sinus rhythm.

If the mitral stenosis is severe then the OS occurs nearer A_2 and the MDM is longer.

Extra points

- **Haemodynamic significance**:
  Pulmonary hypertension: functional tricuspid regurgitation, right ventricular heave, loud P_2.
  Pulmonary oedema.
- **Endocarditis**
- **Embolic complications:** stroke and absent pulses.
- Other rheumatic valve lesions.

Discussion

Causes

Congenital (rare).

Acquired:
  Rheumatic (commonest).
  Senile degeneration.

Differential diagnosis
Left atrial myxoma.
Austin–Flint murmur.

Investigation
- **ECG:** p-mitrale and atrial fibrillation.
- **CXR:** enlarged left atrium, calcified valve and pulmonary oedema.
- **TTE/TOE:** valve area ($< 1\,cm^2$ is critical), cusp mobility and calcification and left atrial thrombus.

Treatment
- **Medical:** Digoxin, Warfarin, diuretics and prophylactic antibiotics.
- **Valvuloplasty:** for pliable non-calcified valves with minimal regurgitation and no left atrial thrombus.
- **Surgery:** closed mitral valvotomy (without opening the heart) or open valvotomy (requiring cardiopulmonary bypass) or valve replacement.

Rheumatic fever
- Immunological cross-reactivity between Group A β-haemolytic streptococcal infection, e.g. *Streptococcus pyogenes* and valve tissue.
- **Duckett–Jones diagnostic criteria**

Proven β-haemolytic streptococcal infection diagnosed by throat swab, ASOT or clinical scarlet fever **plus** 2 major or 1 major and 2 minor:

Major	Minor
Chorea	Raised ESR
Erythema marginatum	Raised WCC
Subcutaneous nodules	Arthralgia
Polyarthritis	Previous rheumatic fever
Carditis	Pyrexia
	Prolonged PR interval

- **Treatment:** Rest, high-dose aspirin and penicillin.
- **Prophylaxis:** monthly penicillin for about 5 yrs.

Mitral incompetence

This patient has been short of breath and tired. Please examine his cardiovascular system.

Clinical signs
- Scars: lateral thoracotomy (valvotomy).
- Pulse: AF, small volume.
- Apex: displaced and volume loaded.
- Palpation: thrill at apex.
- Auscultation:

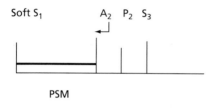

Soft S_1 A_2 P_2 S_3

PSM

Pan-systolic murmur (PSM) loudest at the apex radiating to the axilla. Loudest in expiration. Wide splitting of A_2P_2 due to the earlier closure of A_2 because the LV empties sooner.

S_3 indicates rapid ventricular filling from LA, and excludes significant mitral stenosis.

Extra points
- Pulmonary oedema.
- Endocarditis.
  - Severity: left ventricular failure and atrial fibrillation (late). **Not intensity of the murmur**.
- Other murmurs, e.g. ASD.

Discussion
Causes
- Congenital (associated with secundum ASD).
- Acquired:

	Acute	Chronic
Valve leaflets	Bacterial endocarditis	Rheumatic Connective tissue diseases
Valve annulus		Dilated left ventricle (functional MR) Calcification
Chordae/papillae	Rupture (Post-MI/trauma)	Infiltration, e.g. amyloid

Investigation
- **ECG:** p-mitrale, atrial fibrillation and infarction.
- **CXR:** cardiomegaly and pulmonary oedema.
- **TTE/TOE:**
  Severity: Size of jet and LV systolic function.
  Cause: Vegetations or ruptured papillae.

Management
- **Medical**
  - Anti-coagulation for atrial fibrillation or embolic complications.
  - Diuretic and ACE inhibitors.
  - Antibiotic prophylaxis.
- **Surgical**
  - Valve repair (preferable) or replacement.
  - Aim to operate when symptomatic, prior to severe LV dilatation and dysfunction.

Prognosis
- Often asymptomatic for >10 yrs.
- Mortality 5% per yr in symptomatic patients.

Mitral valve prolapse
- Common (5%), especially young tall women.
- Associated with connective tissue disease, e.g. Marfan's syndrome, and HOCM.
- Often asymptomatic, but may present with chest pain, syncope, palpitations.
- Small risk of emboli and endocarditis (antibiotic prophylaxis required).
- Auscultation:

S_1 EC A_2 P_2 S_3

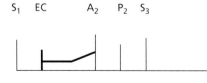

Mid-systolic ejection click (EC). Pan-systolic murmur that gets louder up to A_2.

Murmur is accentuated by standing from a squatting position or during the straining phase of the Valsalva manoeuvre, which reduces the flow of blood through the heart.

Right heart valve abnormalities

Tricuspid incompetence

Examine this patient's cardiovascular system. He has been complaining of abdominal discomfort.

Clinical signs
- Raised JVP with giant CV waves.
- Thrill left sternal edge.
- Auscultation:

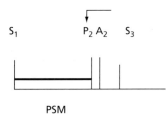

S_1 $P_2 A_2$ S_3

PSM

Pan-systolic murmur (PSM) loudest at the tricuspid area in inspiration.

Reverse split second heart sound due to rapid RV emptying.

Right ventricular rapid filling gives an S_3.

- Pulsatile liver, ascites and peripheral oedema.

Extra points
- Endocarditis from IV drug abuse: needle marks.
- Pulmonary hypertension: RV heave and loud P_2.
- Other valve lesions: rheumatic mitral stenosis.

Discussion
Causes
- **Congenital**: Ebstein's anomaly (atrialization of the right ventricle and TR).
- **Acquired:**
  Acute: infective endocarditis (IV drug user).
  Chronic: functional (commonest), rheumatic and carcinoid syndrome.

Treatment
- **Medical:** diuretics, ACE inhibitors, and support stockings for oedema.
- **Surgical:** valve repair if medical treatment fails.

Pulmonary stenosis

Examine this patient's cardiovascular system. He has had swollen ankles.

Clinical signs
- Raised JVP with giant a waves.
- Left parasternal heave.
- Thrill in the pulmonary area.
- Auscultation:

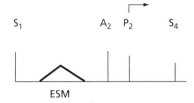

S_1 A_2 P_2 S_4

ESM

Ejection systolic murmur (ESM) heard loudest in the pulmonary area in inspiration.

Widely split second heart sounds, due to a delay in RV emptying.

Severe: inaudible P_2, longer murmur duration obscuring A_2.

Extra points
- Noonan's syndrome: phenotypically like Turner's syndrome but male sex.
- Other valve lesions: functional TR.
- Right ventricular failure: ascites and peripheral oedema.

Discussion
Investigation
- ECG: p-pulmonale, RVH, RBBB.
- CXR: oligaemic lung fields and large right atrium.
- TTE: gradient calculation.

Management
- Pulmonary valvoplasty.
- Pulmonary valvotomy if gradient >70 mmHg or there is RV failure.

Carcinoid syndrome
- Gut primary with liver metastasis secreting 5-HT into the systemic circulation.
- Toilet-symptoms: diarrhoea, wheeze and flushing!
- Secreted mediators scar and thicken the right-sided heart valves resulting in tricuspid regurgitation and/or pulmonary stenosis.
- Rarely a bronchogenic primary tumour can release 5-HT into the systemic circulation and cause left-sided valve scarring.

Prosthetic valves: aortic and mitral

This patient has recently been treated for dyspnoea/chest pain/ syncope. Please examine his cardiovascular system.

Clinical signs
• Audible prosthetic clicks (metal) on approach and scars on inspection:

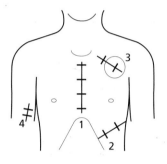

1 Midline sternotomy (CABG, AVR, MVR)
2 Lateral thoracotomy (MVR, mitral valvotomy, coarctation repair, BT shunt)
3 Subclavicular (Pacemaker, AICD)
4 Anticubital fossa (Angiography)

Also look in the groins for angiography scars/bruising and legs for saphenous vein harvest used in bypass grafts.

• Auscultation: don't panic!

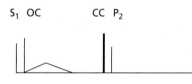

S₁ OC   CC P₂

Flow murmur

Aortic valve replacement

A metal prosthetic closing click (CC) is heard instead of A₂. There may be an opening click (OC) and ejection systolic flow murmur.
A heterograft bioprosthesis (porcine) often has normal heart sounds.

Abnormal findings:
AR
Decreased intensity of the closing click

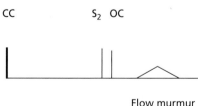

CC   S₂ OC

Flow murmur

Mitral valve replacement

A metal prosthetic closing click is heard instead of S₁. An opening click may be heard in early diastole followed by a low-frequency diastolic rumble. A porcine valve replacement often has normal heart sounds.

Abnormal findings:
MR
Decreased intensity of the closing click.

Extra points
Complications
- Bacterial endocarditis signs.
- Valve failure: see abnormal findings above.
- Anti-coagulation: bruises (metal valve) and anaemia.

Cause
- Multiple valve murmurs/replacements: rheumatic fever.
- Saphenous vein harvest scars: aortic valve replacement more likely.

Discussion
- Choice of valve replacement

	For	Against	Indication
Metal	Durable	Warfarin	Young/On Warfarin, e.g. for AF
Porcine	No Warfarin	Less durable (10 yrs)	Elderly/At risk of haemorrhage

- Operative mortality: 3–5%. Survival @ 10 yrs: 50%.
- Late complications
  - **Thromboembolus:** 1–2% per annum despite warfarin.
  - **Bleeding:** 1% per annum on warfarin.
  - **Prosthetic dysfunction and LVF.**
  - **Haemolysis:** mechanical destruction against the metal valve.
  - **Infective endocarditis:**
    - Early infective endocarditis (<2/12 post-op) can be due to *Staphylococcus epidermidis* from skin.
    - Late infective endocarditis is often due to *Strep. viridans* by haematogenous spread.
    - A second valve replacement is usually required to treat this complication.
    - Mortality of prosthetic valve endocarditis approaches 60%.

Ventricular septal defect

This patient has developed sudden shortness of breath. Examine his heart.

Clinical signs
- Thrill at the left lower sternal edge.
- Auscultation:

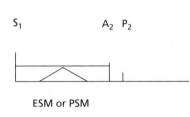

S_1 A_2 P_2

ESM or PSM

Systolic murmur well localized at the left stemal edge with no radiation.
Second heart sounds are often obliterated.

Loudness does not correlate with size (Maladie de Roger: loud murmur due to high-flow velocity through a small VSD).

If Eisenmenger's develops the murmur often disappears as the gradient diminishes.

Extra points
- Other associated lesions: AR, PDA (10%), Fallot's tetralogy, and coarctation.
- Pulmonary hypertension: loud P_2 and RV heave.
- Shunt reversal: right to left (Eisenmenger's syndrome): cyanosis and clubbing.
- Endocarditis.

Discussion
Causes
- Congenital
- Acquired (traumatic or post-MI)

Investigation
- ECG: conduction defect.
- CXR: pulmonary plethora.
- TTE/TOE: site, size and shunt calculation.
- Cardiac catheterization: O_2-saturation measurements quantify shunt size; aortography excludes a PDA and coarctation.

Treatment

Surgical closure of haemodynamically significant lesions.

Associations

1. Fallot's tetralogy

• Right ventricular hypertrophy.
• Overriding aorta.
• VSD.
• Pulmonary stenosis.

Blalock–Taussig shunts

• Corrects the Fallot's abnormality by anastomosing the subclavian artery to the pulmonary artery.
• Causes an absent radial pulse in these patients.

Other causes of an absent radial pulse

• **Acute:** embolism, aortic dissection, trauma, e.g. cardiac catheter, and death(!)
• **Chronic:** coarctation, Takayasu's arteritis ('pulseless disease').

2. Coarctation

A congenital narrowing of the aortic arch that is usually distal to the left subclavian artery.

Clinical signs

• Hypertension in right $\pm$ left arm.
• Prominent upper body pulses, absent/weak femoral pulses, radio-femoral delay.
• Heaving pressure loaded apex.
• Auscultation: continuous murmur from the coarctation and collaterals radiating through to the back. There is a loud A_2. There may be murmurs from associated lesions.

Discussion

Associations:

• **Cardiac:** VSD, bicuspid aortic valve and PDA.
• **Non-cardiac:** Turner's syndrome, and Berry aneurysms.

Investigation:

• ECG: LVH, RBBB.
• CXR: rib notching, double aortic knuckle (post-stenotic dilatation).

Treatment:
- Balloon angioplasty and stent.
- Surgical.
- Long-term anti-hypertensive therapy.

3. Patent ductus arteriosus (PDA)

Continuity between the aorta and pulmonary trunk with left to right shunt.
Risk factor: rubella.

Clinical signs
- Collapsing pulse.
- Thrill second left inter-space.
- Thrusting apex beat.
- Auscultation: loud continuous 'machinery murmur' loudest below the left clavicle in systole.

Discussion
Complications:
- Eisenmenger's reaction (5%).
- Endocarditis.

Treatment: Closed surgically or via cardiac catheter with an occlusion device.

Atrial septal defect

This young woman complains of cough and occasional palpitations. Examine her cardiovascular system.

Clinical signs

- Raised JVP.
- Pulmonary area thrill.
- Auscultation:

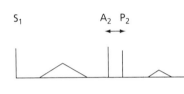

S_1 A_2 P_2

Pulmonary ESM   Tricuspid flow
murmur

Fixed split-second heart sounds that do not change with respiration. Pulmonary ejection systolic flow murmur and tricuspid diastolic flow murmur with large left-to-right shunts.
A loud P_2 indicates pulmonary hypertension.
There is no mumur from the ASD itself.

Extra points

- Pulmonary hypertension: RV heave and loud P_2.
- Congestive cardiac failure.
- Down's syndrome: endocardial cushion defect causes a primum ASD and other atrioventricular valve abnormalities.

Discussion

Types

- Primum (nearest the atrioventricular valve apparatus).
- Secundum (commonest).

Complications

- Paradoxical embolus.
- Atrial arrhythmias.
- Congestive cardiac failure.
- Endocarditis is rare.

Investigation

- ECG: RBBB+LAD (primum) or +RAD (secundum); atrial fibrillation.

- CXR: small aortic knuckle, pulmonary plethora and double-heart-border (enlarged right atrium).
- TTE/TOE: site, size and shunt calculation; amenability to closure.
- Cardiac catheter: shunt calculation.

Management
- Surgical vs. cardiac catheter closure using an 'umbrella' device.

Hypertrophic obstructive cardiomyopathy

This young man has complained of palpitations whilst playing football. Examine his cardiovascular system.

Clinical signs
- Jerky pulse character.
- Double apical impulse (palpable atrial and ventricular contraction).
- Thrill at the lower left sternal edge.
- Auscultation:

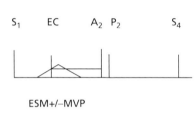

ESM+/–MVP

Ejection systolic murmur (ESM) at the left sternal edge that radiates throughout the precordium. Associated with MVP: ejection click and late systolic murmur.
A fourth heartsound (S_4) is present due to blood hitting a hypertrophied stiff LV during atrial systole.
ESM is accentuated by reducing blood flow through the heart, e.g. standing from a squatting position or straining during a Valsalva manoeuvre.

Extra points
- Associated mitral valve prolapse (MVP).
- Features of Friedreich's ataxia or myotonic dystrophy.
- Family history.

Discussion
Investigation
- ECG: LVH with strain and LAD.
- CXR: often normal.
- TTE: asymmetrical septal hypertrophy and systolic anterior motion of the anterior mitral leaflet on M-mode.
- Genetic tests.

Treatment
- Drugs: B-blockers.
Avoid nitrates and digoxin.
- Dual chamber pacemaker.

- Surgery: Septal myotomy and MVR.
- Alcohol septal ablation.

Prognosis
- Annual mortality rate in adults is 2.5%.
- Poor prognosis factors:
  - Young age at diagnosis.
  - Syncope.
  - Family history of sudden death.

Dystrophia myotonica

This man complains of worsening weakness in his hands. Please examine him.

Clinical signs
Face
- Myopathic facies: long, thin and expressionless.
- Wasting of facial muscles and sternocleidomastoid.
- Bilateral ptosis.
- Frontal balding.
- Dysarthria: due to myotonia of tongue and pharynx.

Hands
- **Myotonia**: 'Grip my hand, now let go' (may be obscured by profound weakness).
  'Screw up your eyes tightly shut, now open them'.
- **Wasting** and **weakness** of distal muscles with areflexia.
- **Percussion myotonia**: percuss thenar eminence and watch for involuntary thumb flexion.

Extra points
- Cataracts.
- Cardiomyopathy, brady- and tachy-arrhythmias (look for pacemaker scar).
- Diabetes (ask to dip urine).
- Testicular atrophy.
- Dysphagia (ask about swallowing).

Discussion
Inheritance
- Autosomal dominant.
- Onset in 20s.
- **Genetic anticipation**: worsening severity of the condition and earlier age of presentation with progressive generations. Due to expansion of tri-nucleotide repeat sequences.

Also occurs in Huntington's chorea (autosomal dominant) and Friedreich's ataxia (autosomal recessive).

Management
- Weakness is major problem—no treatment.
- Phenytoin may help myotonia.
- Advise against general anaesthetic.

Common causes of ptosis

Bilateral	Unilateral
Myotonic dystrophy	Third nerve palsy
Myasthenia gravis	Horner's syndrome
Congenital	

Cerebellar syndrome

*This 37-year-old woman has noticed increasing problems with her
coordination. Please examine her and suggest a diagnosis.*

Clinical signs

Brief conversation	Scanning dysarthria	
Outstretched arms	Rebound phenomenon	
Movements:		
Upper limbs	Finger–nose incoordination	Dysdiadochokinesis
	Hypotonia	Hyporeflexia
Eyes	Nystagmus	
Lower limbs	Heel–shin	Foot tapping
	Wide-based gait	

Extra points

• Direction of nystagmus: clue to the site of the lesion.

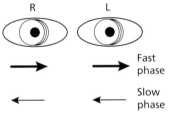

R   L

Fast phase

Slow phase

The direction of the fast phase
determines the direction of
the nystagmus.

Cerebellar lesion
The fast-phase direction is TOWARDS
the side of the lesion, and is maximal
on looking TOWARDS the lesion.

Vestibular nucleus/VIII nerve lesion
The fast-phase direction is AWAY FROM
the side of the lesion, and is maximal
on looking AWAY FROM the lesion.

In this case the nystagmus could be
due to a cerebellar lesion on the LEFT
or a vestibular nucleus lesion on the
RIGHT.

• Cerebellar vermis lesions produce an ataxic trunk and gait but the
limbs are normal when tested on the bed.

• Cerebellar lobe lesions produce **ipsilateral** cerebellar signs in the limbs.

Discussion

Mnemonic for signs

Dysdiadochokinesis
Ataxia
Nystagmus
Intention tremor
Scanning dysarthria
Hypotonia/hyporeflexia

And causes

Posterior fossa tumour
Alcohol
Sclerosis (MS)
Trauma
Rare
Inherited, e.g. Friedreich's ataxia
Epileptic medication
Stroke

Aetiological clues

- Internuclear ophthalmoplegia, spasticity, female, younger age — MS
- Optic atrophy — MS, Friedreich's ataxia
- Clubbing, tar-stained fingers, radiotherapy burn — Bronchial carcinoma
- Stigmata of liver disease, unkempt appearance — EtOH
- Neuropathy — EtOH, Friedrich's ataxia
- Gingival hypertrophy — Phenytoin

Multiple sclerosis

This 30-year-old woman complains of double vision and in-coordination with previous episodes of weakness. Please perform a neurological examination.

Clinical signs
- **Inspection**: ataxic handshake and wheelchair.
- **Cranial nerves**: internuclear ophthalmoplegia (frequently bilateral in MS), optic atrophy, reduced visual acuity, and any other cranial nerve palsy.

Internuclear ophthalmoplegia

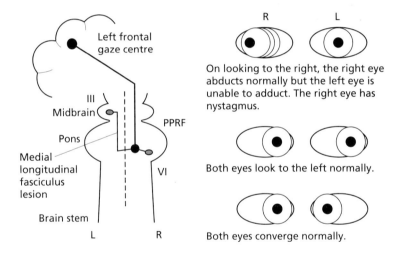

On looking to the right, the right eye abducts normally but the left eye is unable to adduct. The right eye has nystagmus.

Both eyes look to the left normally.

Both eyes converge normally.

- **Peripheral nervous system**: Upper-motor neurone spasticity, weakness, brisk reflexes and altered sensation.
- **Cerebellar**: 'DANISH' (see cerebellar syndrome section).

Extra points
- Higher mental function: euphoria, depression and disinhibition.
- Autonomic: urinary retention/incontinence, impotence and bowel problems.

Discussion
Diagnostic criteria
Central nervous system demyelination (plaques) causing neurological impairment that is disseminated in both **time** and **space**.

Cause
Unknown but genetic susceptibility is evident, e.g. HLA DR2 and possibly environmental factors play a role (increasing incidence with increasing latitude).

Investigation: clinical diagnosis plus
- CSF: oligoclonal IgG bands.
- MRI: periventricular white matter plaques.
- Visual evoked potentials: delayed velocity but normal amplitude.

Treatment
Multidisciplinary approach
Nurse, physiotherapist, occupational therapist, social worker and physician

Disease modifying treatments
- Interferon β and Glatiramer.

Symptomatic treatments
- Methyl-prednisolone during the acute phase may shorten the duration of the 'attack' but does not affect the prognosis.
- Anti-spasmodics, e.g. Baclofen.
- Carbamazepine (for neuropathic pain).
- Laxatives and intermittent catheterization/Oxybutynin for bowel and bladder disturbance.

Prognosis
Variable. The majority will remain ambulant at 10 yrs.

Uthoff's phenomenon: worsening of symptoms after a hot bath or exercise.

Lhermitte's Sign: lightening pains down the spine on neck flexion due to cervical cord plaques.

Impairment, disability and handicap:
- Arm paralysis is the impairment.
- Inability to write is the disability.
- Subsequent inability to work as an accountant is the handicap.

Occupational therapy aim to help minimize the disability and abolish the handicap of arm paresis.

Stroke

Examine this patient's limbs neurologically and then proceed to examine anything else that you feel is important.

Clinical signs

- **Inspection**: walking aides, nasogastric tube or PEG tube, posture (flexed upper limbs and extended lower limbs), wasted or oedematous on affected side.
- **Tone**: spastic rigidity, 'clasp knife' (resistance to movement, then sudden release). Ankles may demonstrate clonus (> 4 beats).
- **Power**: reduced.

MRC graded:

0, none
1, flicker
2, moves with gravity neutralized
3, moves against gravity
4, reduced power against resistance
5, normal

Extensors are usually weaker than flexors in the upper limbs and vice versa in the lower limbs.

- **Coordination**: reduced often due to weakness (but can be seen in posterior circulation strokes).
- **Reflexes**: brisk with extensor plantars.

Offer to

- Walk the patient if they are able to, to demonstrate the flexed posture of the upper limb and 'tip toeing' of the lower limb.
- Test sensation (this is tricky and should be avoided if possible!). Proprioception is important for rehabilitation.

Extra points

- Upper motor neurone unilateral facial weakness (spares frontalis due to its dual innervation).
- Gag reflex and swallow to minimize aspiration.
- Visual fields and higher cortical functions, e.g. neglect helps determine a Bamford classification.
- **Cause**: irregular pulse (AF), blood pressure, cardiac murmurs or carotid bruits (anterior circulation stroke).

Discussion
Definitions
- **Stroke:** rapid onset, focal neurological deficit due to a vascular lesion lasting > 24 h.
- **Transient ischaemic attack (TIA):** focal neurological deficit lasting < 24 h.

Investigation
- **Bloods:** FBC ESR (young CVA may be due to arteritis), glucose, renal function.
- **ECG:** AF or previous infarction.
- **CXR:** cardiomegaly or aspiration.
- **CT head:** infarct or bleed, territory.
- Consider Echo, carotid doppler and clotting screen.

Management
Acute
- **Aspirin.**
- Referral to a specialist stroke unit: **multidisciplinary approach**: physiotherapy, occupational therapy, speech and language therapy and specialist stroke rehabilitation nurses.
- DVT prophylaxis.
- Thrombolysis may be a future possibility but has resource implications.

Chronic (>2/52)
- Carotid endarterectomy in patients who have made a good recovery, e.g. in PACS (>70% stenosis of the ipsilateral internal carotid artery).
- Anti-coagulation for cardiac thromboembolism.
- Address risk factors.
- Nursing care.

Bamford classification of stroke (*Lancet* 1991)
Total anterior circulation stroke (TACS)
- Hemiplegia (contra-lateral to the lesion).
- Homonomous hemianopia (contra-lateral to the lesion).
- Higher cortical dysfunction, e.g. dysphasia, dyspraxia and neglect.

Partial anterior circulation (PACS)
- 2/3 of the above.

Lacunar (LACS)
- Pure hemi-motor or sensory loss.

Prognosis at 1 yr (%)

	TACS	PACS	LACS
Dead	60	15	10
Dependent	35	30	30
Independent	5	55	60

Dominant parietal-lobe cortical signs
- **Dysphasia:** receptive, expressive or global.
- **Gerstmann's syndrome**
  - Dysgraphia, dyslexia and dyscalculia
  - L-R disorientation
  - Finger agnosia

Non-dominant parietal-lobe signs
- Dressing and constructional apraxia.
- Spatial neglect.

Either
- Sensory and visual inattention.
- Astereognosis.
- Graphaesthesia.

Visual field defects

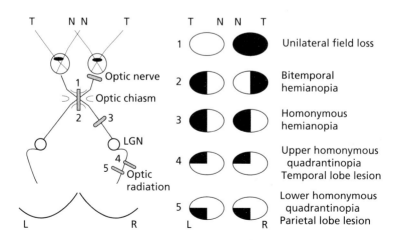

Spastic legs

> *Examine this gentleman's lower limbs neurologically. He has had difficulty in walking.*

Clinical signs

- Wheelchair and walking sticks (disuse atrophy and contractures may be present if chronic).
- Increased tone and ankle clonus.
- Generalized weakness.
- Hyper-reflexia and extensor plantars.
- Gait: 'scissoring'.

Extra points

- Examine for a sensory level suggestive of a spinal lesion.
- Look at the back for scars or spinal deformity.
- Search for features of multiple sclerosis, e.g. cerebellar signs especially dysarthria, fundoscopy to look for optic atrophy.
- Ask about bladder symptoms and note the presence or absence of urinary catheter. **Offer to test anal tone.**

Discussion

Common causes

- Multiple sclerosis.
- Spinal cord compression/cervical myelopathy.
- Trauma.
- Motor neurone disease (no sensory signs).

Other causes

- Anterior spinal artery thrombosis: dissociated sensory loss with preservation of dorsal columns.
- Syringomyelia: with typical upper limb signs.
- Hereditary spastic paraplegia: stiffness exceeds weakness, positive family history.
- Subacute combined degeneration of the cord: absent reflexes with up-going plantars.
- Friedreich's ataxia.
- Parasagittal falx meningioma.

Cord compression

- **Medical emergency.**
- **Causes**

- **Disc prolapse** (above L1/2).
- Malignancy.
- Infection: abscess or TB.
- Trauma: # vertebra.
- **Investigation of choice:** spinal MRI.
- **Treatment**
  - Urgent surgical decompression.
  - Consider steroids and radiotherapy (for a malignant cause).

Lumbo-sacral root levels

L 2/3	Hip flexion	
L 3/4	Knee extension	**Knee jerk L 3/4**
L 4/5	Foot dorsi-flexion	
L 5/S 1	Knee flexion	
	Hip extension	
S 1/2	Foot plantar-flexion	**Ankle jerk S 1/2**

Lower limb dermatomes

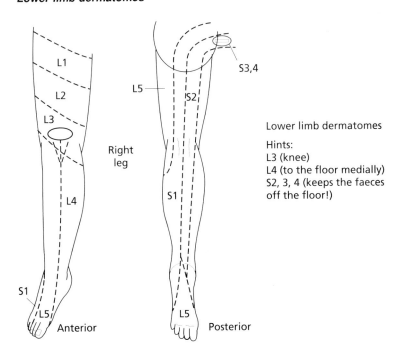

Lower limb dermatomes

Hints:
L3 (knee)
L4 (to the floor medially)
S2, 3, 4 (keeps the faeces off the floor!)

Syringomyelia

Examine this patient's upper limbs neurologically. He has been complaining of numb hands.

Clinical signs
- Weakness and wasting of small muscles of the hand.
- Loss of reflexes in the upper limbs.
- Dissociated sensory loss in upper limbs and chest: loss of pain and temperature sensation (spinothalamic) with preservation of joint position and vibration sense (dorsal columns).
- Scars from painless burns.
- Charcot joints: elbow and shoulder.

Extra points
- Pyramidal weakness in lower limbs with up-going (extensor) plantars.
- Kyphoscoliosis is common.
- Horner's syndrome (see Ophthalmology section).
- If syrinx extends into brain stem (syringobulbia) there may be cerebellar and lower cranial nerve signs.

Discussion
- Syringomyelia is caused by a progressively expanding fluid filled cavity (syrinx) within the cervical cord, typically spanning several levels.

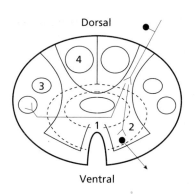

Dorsal

Ventral

Syrinx expands ventrally affecting:

1 Decussating spinothalamic neurones producing segmental pain and temperature loss at the level of the syrinx.

2 Anterior horn cells producing segmental lower motor neurone weakness at the level of the syrinx.

3 Corticospinal tract producing upper motor neurone weakness below the level of the syrinx.

It usually spares the dorsal columns 4 (proprioception).

- The signs may be asymmetrical.

- Frequently associated with an Arnold–Chiari malformation and spina bifida.
- Investigation of choice spinal MRI.

Charcot's joint (neuropathic arthropathy)
- Painless deformity and destruction of a joint with new bone formation following repeated minor trauma secondary to loss of pain sensation.
- The most important causes are
  - Tabes dorsalis: hip and knee.
  - Diabetes: ankle.
  - Syringomyelia: elbow and shoulder.
- Treatment: bisphosphonates can help.

Cervical roots
C 5/6 Elbow flexion and supination **Biceps and supinator jerks C 5/6**
C 7/8 Elbow extension **Triceps jerk C 7/8**
T 1 Finger adduction

Upper limb dermatomes

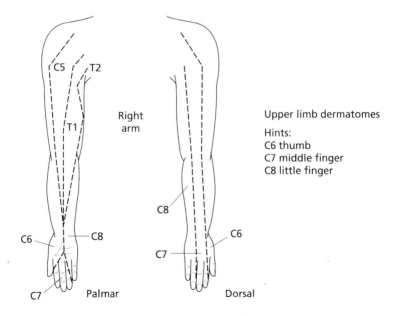

Right arm

Upper limb dermatomes

Hints:
C6 thumb
C7 middle finger
C8 little finger

Palmar

Dorsal

Motor neurone disease

> *This gentleman complains of gradually increasing weakness.*
> *Please examine him neurologically.*

Clinical signs
- **Inspection:** wasting and fasciculation.
- **Tone:** usually spastic but can be flaccid.
- **Power:** weak.
- **Reflexes:** absent and/or brisk. (Absent knee jerk with extensor plantar reflexes.)
- **Sensory examination is normal.**

Extra points
- **Speech:** dysarthria may be bulbar (nasal, 'Donald Duck' speech, due to palatal weakness) or pseudo-bulbar ('hot potato' speech, due to a spastic tongue).
- **Tongue:** wasting and fasciculation (bulbar) or a stiff spastic tongue with brisk jaw jerk (pseudo-bulbar).
- There is no sensory, extra-ocular muscle, cerebellar or extra-pyramidal involvement. Sphincter and cognitive state disturbance is rarely seen.

Discussion
- MND is a progressive disease of unknown aetiology.
- There is axonal degeneration of upper and lower motor neurones.

Motor neurone disease may be classified into three types, although there is often some overlap:
- **Amyotrophic lateral sclerosis** (50%): affecting the cortico-spinal tracts predominantly producing **spastic** paraparesis or tetraparesis.
- **Progressive muscular atrophy** (25%): affecting anterior horn cells predominantly producing wasting, fasciculation and weakness. **Best prognosis.**
- **Progressive bulbar palsy** (25%): affecting lower cranial nerves and supra-bulbar nuclei producing speech and swallow problems. **Worst prognosis.**

Investigation
- Clinical diagnosis.
- **EMG:** fasciculation.
- **MRI:** excludes the main differential diagnosis of cervical cord compression and myelopathy.

Treatment
- Supportive, e.g. PEG feeding and NIPPV.
- Multidisciplinary approach to care.
- Riluzole® (glutamate antagonist): slows disease progression by an average of 3 months but does not improve function or quality of life and is costly.

Prognosis
- Most die within 3 yrs of diagnosis from bronchopneumonia and respiratory failure. Some disease variants may survive longer.
- Worst if elderly at onset, female and with bulbar involvement.

Causes of generalized wasting of hand muscles
- **Anterior horn cell**
  - MND.
  - Syringomyelia.
  - Cervical cord compression.
  - Polio.
- **Brachial plexus**
  - Cervical rib.
  - Pancoast's tumour.
  - Trauma.
- **Peripheral nerve**
  - Combined median and ulnar nerve lesions.
  - Peripheral neuropathy.
- **Muscle**
  - Disuse atrophy, e.g. rheumatoid arthritis.

Fasciculation
- Visible muscle twitching at rest.
- Cause: axonal loss results in the surviving axons recruiting and innervating more myofibrils than usual resulting in large motor units.
- Seen commonly in MND and syringomyelia.

Parkinson's disease

This gentleman complains of a persistent tremor. Examine him neurologically.

Clinical signs
- Expressionless face with an absence of spontaneous movements.
- Coarse tremor. **Pill-rolling.** Characteristically asymmetrical.
- **Bradykinesia** (demonstrated by asking patient to oppose each digit onto thumb in quick succession).
- **Cogwheel rigidity** at wrists (enhanced by asking patient to tap with opposite hand on his knee).
- Gait is shuffling and festinates. Absence of arm swinging—often asymmetrical.
- Speech is slow, faint and monotonous.

Extra points
- **BP** looking for evidence of **multisystem atrophy**: Parkinsonism with postural hypotension, cerebellar and pyramidal signs.
- Test **vertical eye movements** (up and down) for evidence of **progressive supranuclear palsy.**
- **Dementia** and Parkinsonism: **Lewy-body dementia.**
- Ask for a **medication** history.

Discussion
Causes of Parkinsonism
Parkinson's disease (idiopathic)
Parkinson Plus syndromes:
   Multisystem Atrophy (Shy–Drager)
   Progressive Supranuclear Palsy (Steel–Richardson–Olszewski)
Drug-induced, particularly phenothiazines
Anoxic brain damage
Post-encephalitis
MPTP toxicity ('frozen addict syndrome')

Pathology
- Degeneration of the dopaminergic neurones between the substantia nigra and basal ganglia.

Treatment
- **Dopamine agonists**, e.g. Pergolide.

- **MAO-B inhibitor**, e.g. Selegiline, inhibit the breakdown of dopamine.
- Anti-cholinergics are effective for reducing tremor, particularly drug-induced.
- **Apomorphine** given as an SC injection or infusion.
- L-**Dopa** with a peripheral Dopa-decarboxylase inhibitor, e.g. Madopar.
  - Problems with nausea and dyskinesia.
  - Effects wear off after a few years so generally delay treatment as long as possible.
  - End of dose effect and on/off motor fluctuation may be reduced by modified release preparations.
- **COMT inhibitors**, e.g. Entacapone, block breakdown of L-Dopa outside the brain thus reducing motor fluctuations.
- **Surgery:** thalamotomy, pallidotomy, deep brain stimulation and fetal neural transplantation.

Causes of tremor
- **Resting tremor:** Parkinson's disease
- **Postural tremor** (worse with arms outstretched):
  - Benign essential tremor (50% familial) improves with EtOH.
  - Anxiety.
  - Thyrotoxicosis.
  - Metabolic: CO_2 and hepatic encephalopathy.
  - Alcohol.
- **Intention tremor**: seen in cerebellar disease.

Hereditary sensory motor neuropathy

This gentleman complains his legs have begun to look unusual over the last few years. Please examine him neurologically.

Clinical signs
- Wasting of distal lower limb muscles with preservation of the thigh muscle bulk (inverted champagne bottle appearance).
- Pes cavus (seen also in Friedreich's ataxia).
- Weakness of ankle dorsi-flexion and toe extension.
- Variable degree of stocking distribution sensory loss (usually mild).

Extra points
- Gait is high stepping (due to foot drop) and stamping (absent proprioception).
- Wasting of hand muscles.
- Palpable lateral popliteal nerve.

Discussion
- The commonest HSMN types are I (demyelinating) and II (axonal).
- Autosomal dominant inheritance.
- HSMN is also known as Charcot–Marie–Tooth disease and peroneal muscular atrophy.

Other causes of peripheral neuropathy
Predominantly sensory
- Diabetes mellitus.
- Alcohol.
- Drugs, e.g. Isoniazid and Vincristine.
- Vitamin deficiency, e.g. B_{12} and B_1.

Predominantly motor
- Guillain–Barré and Botulism present acutely.
- Lead toxicity.
- Porphyria.
- HSMN.

Mononeuritis multiplex
- Diabetes mellitus.
- Connective tissue disease, e.g. SLE and rheumatoid arthritis.
- Vasculitis, e.g. Polyarteritis nodosa and Churg–Strauss.
- Infection, e.g. HIV.
- Malignancy.

Friedreich's ataxia

Examine this young man's neurological system.

Clinical signs
- Young adult, wheelchair.
- Pes cavus.
- Bilateral cerebellar ataxia (ataxic hand shake).
- Pyramidal leg weakness (bilateral extensor plantars).
- Peripheral neuropathy with muscle wasting and loss of ankle and knee jerks.
- Posterior column signs (loss of vibration and joint position sense).

Extra points
- Cerebellar signs in the arms, nystagmus and scanning dysarthria.
- Kyphoscoliosis.
- Optic atrophy (30%).
- Sensi-neural deafness (10%).
- Listen for murmur of HOCM.
- Ask to dip urine (10% develop diabetes).

Discussion
- Inheritance is usually autosomal recessive.
- Onset is during teenage years.
- Survival rarely exceeds 20 yrs from diagnosis.
- There is an association with HOCM and a mild dementia.

Causes of extensor plantars with absent knee jerks
- Friedreich's ataxia.
- Subacute combined degeneration of the cord.
- Motor neurone disease.
- Taboparesis.
- Conus medullaris lesions.
- Combined upper and lower pathology, e.g. cervical spondylosis with peripheral neuropathy.

Facial nerve palsy

Examine this patient's cranial nerves. What is wrong?

Clinical signs
- Unilateral facial droop, absent nasolabial fold and forehead creases.
- Inability to raise the eyebrows (frontalis), screw the eyes up (orbicularis oculi) or smile (orbicularis oris).

Bell's phenomenon: eyes roll backwards on attempting to close the eyes.

Extra points
Level of the lesion
• **Pons**	+VI palsy and long tract signs
MS, stroke	
• **Cerebellar-pontine angle**	+V, VI, VIII and cerebellar signs
Tumour, e.g. acoustic neuroma	
• **Auditory/facial canal**	+VIII
Cholesteatoma, abscess	
• **Neck and face**	+ scars or parotid mass
Tumour, trauma	

Discussion
Commonest cause is Bell's palsy
- Rapid onset (1–2 days).
- HSV-1 has been implicated.
- Induced swelling and compression of the nerve within the facial canal causes demyelination and temporary conduction block.
- Treatment: the role of steroid and Aciclovir is debated.
- **Remember eye protection.**
- Prognosis: 85% make a full recovery.

Other causes of a VII nerve palsy
- Herpes zoster (Ramsay–Hunt syndrome).
- Mononeuropathy due to diabetes, sarcoidosis or Lyme disease.
- Tumour/Trauma.
- MS/stroke.

Causes of bilateral facial palsy
- Guillain–Barré.
- Lyme disease.
- Bilateral Bell's palsy.
- Sarcoidosis.
- Myasthenia gravis.

Myasthenia gravis

"Examine this patient's cranial nerves. She has been suffering with double vision."

Clinical signs
- Bilateral ptosis (worse on sustained upward gaze).
- Complicated bilateral extra-ocular muscle palsies.
- Myasthenic snarl (on attempting to smile).
- Nasal speech, palatal weakness and poor swallow (bulbar involvement).

Extra points
- Demonstrate proximal muscle weakness in the upper limbs and **fatigability.** The reflexes are normal.
- Look for sternotomy scars (thymectomy).

Discussion
- **Associations:** other autoimmune diseases, e.g. diabetes mellitus, rheumatoid arthritis, thyrotoxicosis and SLE, and thymomas.
- **Cause:** Anti-nicotinic acetylcholine receptor antibodies affect motor end-plate neurotransmission.

Investigations
Diagnostic tests
- Edrophonium (Tensilon®) test: an acetylcholine esterase inhibitor increases the concentration of ACh at the motor end plate and hence improves the muscle weakness. **Can cause heart block and even asystole.**

Cholinergic crisis: SLUDGES
Salivation
Lacrimation
Urination
Diarrhoea
Gastric
Emesis
Small pupils
(The brain sludges too, they are confused!).
- Acetylcholine receptor antibodies are present in 90% of cases.
- EMG: decremented response to a titanic train of impulses.

Other tests
- Vital capacity (10% require invasive ventilation).
- CT or MRI of the mediastinum.

Treatments
Acute
- IV immunoglobulin or plasmapheresis.

Chronic
- Acetylcholine esterase inhibitor, e.g. Pyridostigmine.
- Immunosuppression: steroids and Azathioprine.
- Thymectomy is beneficial even if the patient does not have a thymoma (usually young females).

Lambert–Eaton myasthenic syndrome (LEMS)
- Diminished reflexes that become brisker after exercise.
- Lower limb girdle weakness (unlike myasthenia gravis).
- Associated with malignancy, e.g. small-cell lung cancer.
- Antibodies block pre-synaptic calcium channels.
- EMG shows a 'second wind' phenomenon on repetitive stimulation.

Causes of bilateral extra-ocular palsies
- Myasthenia gravis.
- Graves' disease.
- Mitochondrial cytopathies, e.g. Kearns–Sayre syndrome.
- Miller–Fischer variant of Guillain–Barré syndrome.
- Cavernous sinus pathologies.

Causes of bilateral ptosis
- Congenital.
- Senile.
- Myasthenia gravis.
- Myotonic dystrophy.
- Mitochondrial cytopathies, e.g. Kearns–Sayre syndrome.
- Bilateral Horner's syndrome.

Abdominal and Respiratory

Chronic liver disease and hepatomegaly

This gentleman complains of weight loss and abdominal discomfort. His GP has referred him to you for a further opinion. Please examine his abdomen.

Clinical signs
Signs of chronic liver disease
- **General:** Cachexia, icterus (also in acute), excoriation and bruising.
- **Hands:** Leuconychia, clubbing, Dupuytren's contractures and palmar erythema.
- **Face:** Xanthelasma, parotid swelling and fetor hepaticus.
- **Chest and abdomen:** Spider naevi and caput medusa, reduced body hair, gynaecomastia and testicular atrophy (in males).

Signs of hepatomegaly
- Palpation and percussion
  - Mass in the right upper-quadrant that moves with respiration, that you are not able to get above and is dull to percussion.
  - Estimate size (finger breadths below the diaphragm).
  - Smooth or craggy/nodular (malignancy/cirrhosis)
  - Pulsatile (TR in CCF)
- Auscultation
  - Bruit over liver (hepatocellular carcinoma).

Extra points
Evidence of an underlying cause of hepatomegaly
- Tattoos and needle marks   Infectious hepatitis/alcohol
- Pigmentation   Haemochromatosis
- Cachexia   Malignancy
- Mid-line sternotomy scar   CCF

Evidence of treatment
- Ascitic drain/tap sites and peritono-venous shunts.
- Surgical scars.

Evidence of decompensation
- **A**scites: shifting dullness.
- **A**sterixis: 'liver flap'.
- **A**ltered consciousness: encephalopathy.

Discussion
Causes of hepatomegaly
The **Big Three**:
Cirrhosis (early stages)
Carcinoma (secondaries)
Congestive cardiac failure
Plus: Infectious (HBV, HCV)
                Immune (PBC)
                Infiltrative (Amyloid)

Investigations
- Bloods: FBC, clotting, U+E, LFT and glucose.
- Ultrasound scan abdomen.
- Tap ascites (if present).

If cirrhotic
- Liver screen bloods
  - Ferritin (haemochromatosis).
  - Caeruloplasmin (Wilson's disease).
  - α-1 antitrypsin
  - Autoantibodies and immunoglobulins (PBC and autoimmune hepatitis).
  - Hepatitis B and C serology.
  - AFP (hepatocellular carcinoma).
- Hepatic synthetic function: INR (acute) and albumin (chronic).
- Liver biopsy (diagnosis and staging).

If malignancy
- Imaging: CXR and CT abdomen/chest.
- Colonoscopy/Gastroscopy.
- Biopsy.

Complications of cirrhosis
- Variceal haemorrhage due to portal hypertension.
- Hepatic encephalopathy.
- Spontaneous bacterial peritonitis.

Causes of ascites
- Cirrhosis (80%).
- Carcinomatosis.
- CCF.

Treatment of ascites in cirrhotics
- Abstinence from alcohol.
- Salt restriction.
- Diuretics (aim: 1 kg weight loss/day).
- (Liver transplantation).

Causes of palmar erythema
- Cirrhosis.
- Hyperthyroidism.
- Rhematoid arthritis.
- Pregnancy.
- Polycythaemia.

Causes of gynaecomastia
- Physiological: puberty and senility.
- Kleinfelter's syndrome.
- Cirrhosis.
- Drugs, e.g. spironolactone and digoxin.
- Testicular tumour/orchidectomy.
- Endocrinopathy, e.g. hyper/hypothyroidism, Addison's.

Haemochromatosis

This 52-year-old man was referred after a diagnosis of diabetes mellitus was made by his GP. Please examine him and discuss further investigations.

Clinical signs
- Increased skin pigmentation.
- Stigmata of chronic liver disease.
- Hepatomegaly.

Extra points
Scars
- Venesection.
- Liver biopsy.
- Joint replacement.
- Abdominal rooftop incision (hemihepatectomy for hepatocellular carcinoma).

Evidence of complications
- **Endocrine:** 'bronze diabetes'(e.g. injection sites), hypogonadism and testicular atrophy.
- **Cardiac:** congestive cardiac failure.
- **Joints:** arthropathy (pseudo-gout).

Discussion
Inheritance
- Autosomal recessive, chromosome 6.
- **HFE** gene mutation: regulator of gut iron absorption.
- Homozygous prevalence 1 : 300, carrier rate 1 : 10.
- Males affected at an earlier age due to female protective iron loss by menstruation.

Presentation
- Fatigue and arthritis.
- Chronic liver disease.
- Incidental diagnosis or family screening.

Investigation
- ↑ Serum ferritin.

- ↑ Transferrin saturation.
- ↓ Total iron-binding capacity.
- Liver biopsy (diagnosis + staging).
- Genotyping.

And consider

- Blood glucose — Diabetes
- ECG, CXR, ECHO — Cardiac failure
- Liver ultrasound, α-fetoprotein — Hepatocellular carcinoma (HCC)

Treatment

- Regular venesection (1 unit/week) until iron deficient, then venesect 3–4×/yr.
- Avoid alcohol.
- Surveillance for HCC.

Family screening (1st degree relatives aged > 20 yrs)

- Iron studies.

If positive:

- Liver biopsy.
- Genotype analysis.

Prognosis

- 200 × increased risk of HCC if cirrhotic.
- Reduced life expectancy if cirrhotic.
- Normal life expectancy without cirrhosis + effective treatment.

Liver transplantation in haemochromatosis

- Only 50% 1-yr survival.
- High mortality: cardiac + infectious complications.

Splenomegaly

This gentleman presents with tiredness and lethargy. Please examine his abdominal system and discuss your diagnosis.

Clinical signs
General
- Anaemia.
- Lymphadenopathy (axillae, cervical and inguinal areas).
- Purpura.

Abdominal
- Left upper quadrant mass that moves inferomedially with respiration, has a notch, is dull to percussion and you cannot get above nor ballot.
- Estimate size.
- Check for hepatomegaly.

Extra points
- Lymphadenopathy   Haematological, infective
- Stigmata of chronic liver disease   Cirrhosis with portal hypertension
- Splinter haemorrhages,   Bacterial endocarditis
  murmur, etc.
- Rheumatoid hands   Felty's syndrome

Discussion
Causes
- Massive splenomegaly (>8 cm)
  - Myeloproliferative disorders (**CML**).
  - **Myelofibrosis.**
  - Tropical infections (**malaria**, visceral leishmaniasis: **kala-azar**).
- Moderate (4–8 cm)
  - Myelo/lymphoproliferative disorders.
  - Infiltration (Gaucher's and amyloidosis).
- Tip (<4 cm)
  - Myelo/lymphoproliferative disorders.
  - Portal hypertension.
  - Infections (EBV, infective endocarditis, infective hepatitis).
  - Haemolytic anaemia.

Investigations
Ultrasound abdomen
Then if:

- **Haematological**
  - FBC.
  - Blood film.
  - Bone marrow aspirate and trephine.
  - Lymph node biopsy.
- **Infectious**
  - Thick and thin films (malaria).
  - Viral serology.

Indications for splenectomy

- Rupture (trauma).
- Haematological (ITP, hereditary spherocytosis).

Splenectomy work-up

- Vaccination (ideally 2/52 prior to protect against encapsulated bacteria)
  - Pneumococcus.
  - Meningococcus.
  - Haemophilus influenzae (Hib).
- Prophylactic penicillin.
- Medic alert bracelet.

Renal enlargement

> *This lady has been referred by her GP for investigation of hypertension. Please examine her abdomen.*

Clinical signs
Peripheral
- Blood pressure: **hypertension**.
- Arteriovenous fistulae (thrill and bruit).
- Immunosuppressant 'stigmata', e.g. gum hypertrophy with ciclosporin.

Abdomen
- Palpable kidney: ballotable, can get above it and moves with respiration.
- Iliac fossae: scar with (or without!) transplanted kidney.
- Ask to dip the urine: proteinuria and haematuria.
- Ask to examine the external genitalia (varicocele in males).

Extra points
- Hepatomegaly: polycystic kidney disease.
- Indwelling catheter: obstructive nephropathy with hydronephrosis.
- CAPD catheter/scars.

Discussion
Causes of unilateral enlargement
- Simple cysts.
- Renal cell carcinoma.
- Polycystic kidney disease (with unilateral nephrectomy).
- Hydronephrosis (due to ureteric obstruction).

Causes of bilateral enlargement
- Polycystic kidney disease.
- Bilateral renal cell carcinoma (5%).
- Bilateral hydronephrosis.
- Amyloidosis.

Investigations
- U+E.
- Urine cytology.
- Ultrasound abdomen ± biopsy.
- IVU.

- CT if carcinoma is suspected.
- Genetic studies (ADPKD).

Autosomal Dominant Polycystic Kidney Disease
- Progressive cystic degeneration leading to renal failure.
- Incidence 1 : 1000.
- Present with:
  - Hypertension.
  - Recurrent UTIs.
  - Abdominal pain.
  - Haematuria.
- End-stage renal failure by age 40–60 yrs.
- Genetic counselling of family and family screening.
- Treatment: nephrectomy/dialysis/renal transplant.

The transplant patient

Please examine this gentleman's abdomen.

Clinical signs
- Scars:

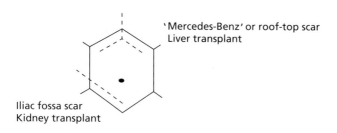

'Mercedes-Benz' or roof-top scar
Liver transplant

Iliac fossa scar
Kidney transplant

Liver
- Evidence of chronic liver disease.

Renal
- Palpate the scar for underlying transplanted kidney: they can be removed again!
- Unilateral/bilateral palpable kidneys.
- Other scars: nephrectomy and/or CAPD catheter.
- Fistulae (usually brachioradial).

Extra points
Reason for liver transplantation
- Pigmentation   Haemochromatosis
- Other autoimmune disease   PBC
- Tattoos, needle marks   Hepatitis B, C

Evidence of immunosuppressive medication
- Ciclosporin: Gum hypertrophy, hypertension.
- Steroids: Cushingoid appearance, thin skin, ecchymoses, etc.

Skin signs
- **Malignancy** (especially renal transplant recipients)

- Dysplastic change (actinic keratoses).
- Squamous cell carcinoma (100 × increased risk, multiple lesions).
- Basal cell carcinoma, malignant melanoma (10 × increased risk).
- **Infection**
  - Viral warts.
  - Cellulitis.

Discussion

Top 3 causes for renal transplantation
- Diabetic nephropathy.
- Glomerulonephritis.
- Polycystic kidney disease (ADPKD).

Top 3 reasons for liver transplantation
- Cirrhosis.
- Acute hepatic failure (hepatitis A and B, Paracetamol overdose).
- Hepatic malignancy.

Problems following transplantation
- **Rejection**
  - Acute (5–10 days): reversible with immunosuppression.
  - Chronic (>6 weeks).
- **Infection secondary to immunosuppression**
  - *Pneumocystis carinii*.
  - CMV.
- **Increased risk of other pathologies**
  - Skin malignancy.
  - Lymphoma.
  - Hypertension and hyperlipidaemia leading to MI and stroke.
- **Immunosuppressant drug side effects/toxicity**
  - Ciclosporin nephrotoxicity.
- **Recurrence of original disease**.
- **Psychological**.

Success of renal transplantation
- 90% 1-yr graft survival.
- 50% 10-yr graft survival (best with live-related donor grafts).

Success of liver transplantation
- 80% 1-yr survival.
- 70% 5-yr survival.

Renal bone disease in patients with chronic renal failure
- **Hyperparathyroidism**
  - Bony reabsorption, osteoporosis and 'telescopic shortening' of phalanges.
  - Parathyroidectomy scars.
- **Osteomalacia**
  - Proximal myopathy.
  - Old fracture sites.
- **Extraskeletal calcification**
  - Periarticular soft tissues (swollen interphalangeal joints).
  - Red-eyes: band keratopathy (conjunctival precipitation).

Causes of gum hypertrophy
- Drugs: Ciclosporin, Phenytoin and Nifedipine.
- Scurvy.
- Acute myelomonocytic leukaemia.
- Pregnancy.
- Familial.

Inflammatory bowel disease

This 36-year-old male has been referred for investigation of bloody diarrhoea. Please examine his abdominal system.

Clinical signs
General
- Pallor/anaemia.
- Slim build.
- Oral ulceration.

Abdomen
- Surgical scars, including current/past stoma sites.
- Tenderness.
- Palpable masses (e.g. right iliac fossa mass in Crohn's disease or colonic tumour in UC).
- Ask to examine for perianal disease.

Extra points
- Evidence of treatment
  - Steroid side-effects.
  - Ciclosporin (gum hypertrophy and hypertension).
  - Hickman lines/scars.
- Extra-intestinal manifestations (see below).

Discussion
Cause
Unknown.

Differential diagnosis
- **Crohn's:** *Yersinia*, tuberculosis, lymphoma (and UC).
- **UC:** infection (e.g. campylobacter), ischaemia, drugs and radiation (and Crohn's).

Investigation
- **Stool microscopy and culture**: exclude infective cause of diarrhoea.
- **FBC, inflammatory markers**: monitor disease activity.
- **AXR**: exclude toxic dilatation in UC and small bowel obstruction due to strictures in Crohn's.
- **Sigmoidoscopy/colonoscopy and biopsy**: histological confirmation.
- **Bowel contrast studies**: strictures, fistulae in Crohn's disease.

- Further imaging: **white cell scan, CT scan**.

Treatment
Medical

• **Drugs**	**Crohn's**	**UC**
Mild-moderate disease	Oral steroid	Oral or topical (rectal steroid)
	(5-ASA)	5-ASA (e.g. mesalazine)
Severe disease	IV steroid	IV steroid
		IV Ciclosporin
Maintenance therapy	Oral steroid	Oral steroid
	Azathioprine	5-ASA
	Methotrexate	
	Infliximab	

- **Nutritional support:** high fibre, elemental and low residue diets.
- **Psychological support.**

Surgery
- **Crohn's:** obstruction from strictures, complications from fistulae and perianal disease and failure to respond to medical therapy.
- **UC:** chronic symptomatic relief, emergency surgery for severe refractory colitis and colonic dysplasia or carcinoma.

Prognosis
- Most lead a normal healthy life once treated with no overall increase in mortality.

Complications

Crohn's disease	Ulcerative colitis
Malabsorption	Anaemia
Anaemia	Toxic dilatation
Abscess	Perforation
Fistula	Colonic carcinoma
Intestinal obstruction	

Colonic carcinoma and UC
- Higher risk in patients with pancolitis: 5–10% at 15–20 yrs.
- Surveillance: 2-yearly colonoscopy for patients with pancolitis >10 yrs is usually recommended.
- Colectomy if dysplasia is detected.

Extra-intestinal manifestations
- **Mouth:**   Apthous ulcers*
- **Skin:**   Erythema nodosum*
  Pyoderma gangrenosum*
- **Joint:**   Large joint arthritis*
  Seronegative arthritides
- **Eye:**   Uveitis*, episcleritis*, conjunctivitis*
- **Liver:**   Primary sclerosing cholangitis (UC)

(* related to disease activity).

Pleural effusion

This patient has been breathless for 2 weeks. Examine his respiratory system to elucidate the cause.

Clinical signs
- Reduced expansion.
- Tracheal or mediastinal (apex beat) displaced away from the side of the effusion.
- **Stony** dull percussion note.
- Reduced vocal resonance and tactile vocal fremitus.
- Reduced air entry and breath sounds.
- Bronchial breathing above.

Extra points
Signs that may indicate the cause
- **Cancer:** clubbing and lymphadenopathy.
- **Congestive cardiac failure:** raised JVP.
- **Chronic liver disease:** leuconychia, spider naevi and gynaecomastia.
- **Chronic renal failure:** arterio-venous fistula.
- **Connective tissue disease:** rheumatoid hands.
- Signs of DVT.

Causes of a dull lung base
- **Consolidation:** bronchial breathing, increased breath sounds and crackles.
- **Collapse:** tracheal deviation towards the side of collapse and reduced breath sounds.
- **Pleural thickening:** signs are similar to a pleural effusion but with normal vocal resonance.
- **Raised hemidiaphragm.**

Discussion
Causes

Transudate (protein <30 g/L)	Exudate (protein >30 g/L)
Congestive cardiac failure	Neoplasm: 1° or 2°
Chronic renal failure	Infection
Chronic liver failure	Infarction
	Inflammation: RA and SLE

Investigation
CXR
- No mediastinal shift indicates collapse as well and a bronchoscopy is indicated.

Pleural aspiration
- **Exudate**
  - **Protein:** effusion albumin/plasma albumin >0.5 (Light's Criteria).
  - **LDH:** effusion LDH/plasma LDH >0.6.
- **Empyema:** an exudate with a low glucose and pH <7.2 is suggestive.

Investigating an exudate (diagnostic percentage)
Pleural fluid cytology (60%),
   plus pleural biopsy (70%),
   plus thoracoscopy (90+%).
CT scan of the thorax may also be useful.

Treatment
Transudate
- Treat the cause.

Exudate
- Intercostal drainage.
- Consider chemical pleurodesis with talc or tetracycline or surgical pleurectomy for recurrent effusions.

Empyema
- A collection of pus within the pleural space.
- Most frequent organisms: anaerobes, staphylococci and Gram-negative organisms.
- Associated with bronchial obstruction, e.g. carcinoma.

Treatment
- Pleural drainage and IV antibiotics.
- Intrapleural streptokinase.
- Surgery.

Bronchiectasis

This 60-year-old woman presents to your clinic with a chronic cough. Please examine her and discuss your findings.

Clinical signs

General: Cachexia and tachypnoea.

Hands: Clubbing.

Chest: Hyperexpanded with mixed character crackles and wheeze. Sputum + + + (look in the pot!). Reduced PEFR.

Extra points

- **Cor pulmonale:** SOA, raised JVP and RV heave.
- **Cause:** lymph nodes elsewhere.

Discussion
Differential diagnosis

- Fibrosing alveolitis
- Bronchial carcinoma
- Lung abscess

Differential diagnosis of CLUBBING + CRACKLES

Investigation

- Sputum culture and cytology.
- CXR: tramlines and ring shadows.
- **High-resolution** CT thorax ('signet ring' sign: thickened, dilated bronchi larger than the adjacent vascular bundle).

For a specific cause

- **Bronchoscopy:** malignancy.
- **Immunoglobulins:** hypogammaglobulinaemia (especially IgG_2 and IgA).
- **Aspergillus precipitins and skin prick testing:** ABPA.
- **Saccharine ciliary motility test** (nares to taste buds in 30 min): Kartagener's.

Causes of bronchiectasis

- **Congenital:** Kartagener's and cystic fibrosis.
- **Mechanical:** bronchial carcinoma (suspect if localized bronchiectasis).
- **Childhood infection:** measles and TB.
- **Immune OVER activity:** allergic broncho-pulmonary aspergillosis (ABPA).

- **Immune UNDER activity:** hypogammaglobulinaemia.
- **Aspiration:** chronic alcoholics.

Treatment
- **Physiotherapy.**
- Antibiotic therapy for exacerbations.
- Longer-term rotating antibiotics.
- Bronchodilators if there is any airflow obstruction.
- Surgery is occasionally used for localized disease.

Complications of bronchiectasis
- Cor pulmonale.
- (Secondary) amyloidosis.
- Massive haemoptysis.
- Metastatic infection, e.g. cerebral abscess.

Cryptogenic fibrosing alveolitis

Examine this patient's respiratory system, she has been complaining of progressive shortness of breath.

Clinical signs
- Clubbing, central cyanosis and tachypnoea.
- Fine end-inspiratory crackles (like Velcro®).
- No sputum.

Extra points
- Signs of associated autoimmune diseases, e.g. rheumatoid arthritis (hands), SLE and systemic sclerosis (face and hands) and Crohn's (mouth ulcers).
- Signs of treatment, e.g. Cushingoid from steroids.

Discussion
Investigation
- **Bloods:** ESR, rheumatoid factor, ANA.
- **CXR:** bilateral basal reticulo-nodular changes.
- **ABG:** type I respiratory failure (low Pao_2 and $Paco_2$).
- **Lung function tests**
  - $FEV_1/FVC > 0.8$ (restrictive)
  - Reduced K_{CO}
- **Broncho-alveolar lavage:** lymphocytes > neutrophils indicate a better response to steroids and a better prognosis.
- **High resolution CT scan**: distribution of fibrosis to peri-pleural lung is typical.
- Lung biopsy.

Treatment
- Immunosuppression, e.g. steroids, but the evidence that any treatment works is weak.
- Single lung transplant (rare).

Prognosis
- 50% mortality at 2 yrs (better if steroid responders).
- There is an increased risk of bronchogenic carcinoma.

Hamman–Rich syndrome
- A rapidly progressive and fatal variant of CFA.

Causes of basal fibrosis

- CFA.
- Asbestosis.
- Drugs: Amiodarone.
- Connective tissue diseases.
- Aspiration.

Old tuberculosis

Please examine this man's respiratory system.

Clinical signs
- Chest deformity and absent ribs.
- Tracheal deviation towards the side of the fibrosis (traction).
- Reduced expansion.
- Dull percussion.
- Crackles and bronchial breathing.

Extra points
- Scars
  - Thoracoplasty.
  - Supraclavicular fossa: phrenic nerve crush.
- Kyphosis: Pott's fracture.

Discussion
- Prior to the development of chemotherapy, inducing apical collapse treated TB. It was thought that the subsequent lower O_2 tension would inhibit TB proliferation.
- Techniques
  - **Plombage:** insertion of polystyrene balls into the thoracic cavity.
  - **Phrenic nerve crush:** diaphragm paralysis.
  - **Thoracoplasty:** rib removal.
- Streptomycin was introduced in the 1950s. It was the first drug shown to be beneficial in a randomized controlled trial.

New treatments involve combination chemotherapy to avoid resistance.

Serious side effects
- **Isoniazid**   peripheral neuropathy (Rx Pyridoxine) and hepatitis.
- **Rifampicin**   hepatitis and increased contraceptive pill metabolism.
- **Ethambutol**   retro-bulbar neuritis.
- **Pyrazinamide**   hepatitis.

Prior to treating TB, check baseline liver function tests and visual acuity, and warn the patient about contraceptive pill failure, urine discoloration and the importance of compliance. They must return immediately if they have visual disturbance.

Complications of old TB
- Aspergilloma in the old TB cavity ± haemoptysis.

- Bronchiectasis due to lymph node compression of large airways and traction from fibrosis.
- Pleural effusion/thickening.
- Scarring from TB predisposes to bronchial carcinoma.

Causes of apical fibrosis TRASHE

- **T**B.
- **R**adiation.
- **A**nkylosing spondylitis.
- **S**arcoidosis.
- **H**istoplasmosis.
- **E**xtrinsic allergic alveolitis.

Pneumonia

This patient has been acutely unwell for 3 days, with shortness of breath and a productive cough. Please examine his chest.

Clinical signs
- Tachypnoea (count respiratory rate), O_2 mask, sputum pot (rusty sputum indicates *pneumococcus*).
- Reduced expansion and increased tactile vocal fremitus.
- Dull percussion note.
- Focal coarse crackles, increased vocal resonance and bronchial breathing.
- Ask for the temperature chart.

Extra points
- Confusion and hypotension are markers of severity.
- Complications, e.g. para-pneumonic effusion.
- Clubbing may indicate an abscess.
- Erythema multiforme: target lesions (*mycoplasma*).

Discussion
Investigation
- **CXR**: consolidation (air bronchogram), abscess, and effusion.
- **Bloods**: WCC, CRP, urea, atypical serology (on admission and at day 10), immunoglobulins.
- **Blood** (25% positive) and **sputum cultures**.
- **Urine:**
  Legionella antigen (in severe cases).
  Pneumococcal antigen.
  Haemoglobinuria (*mycoplasma* causes cold agglutinins → haemolysis).

Management
- O_2.
- Antibiotics.

Community acquired pneumonia (CAP)
- Common organisms
  - *Strep. pneumoniae* 50%.
  - *Mycoplasma pneumoniae* 6%.
  - *Haemophilus influenzae* (especially if COPD).
  - *Chlamydia pneumoniae*.

- Antibiotics
  - 1st line: Penicillin *or* Cephalosporin + Macrolide

Hospital-acquired pneumonia

- Common organisms as above plus
  - *Pseudomonas.*
  - *Staph. aureus.*
  - Gram-negative bacilli.
- Antibiotics
  - 1st line: anti-pseudomonal Penicillin *or* broad spectrum Cephalosporin ± Gentamicin

Special considerations

- **Immunosuppressed**
  - Fungal   Rx Amphotericin
  - Multi-resistant mycobacteria
  - *Pneumocystis carinii*   Rx Cotrimoxazole/Pentamidine
  - CMV   Rx Ganciclovir
- **Aspiration** (commonly posterior segment of right lower lobe)
  - Anaerobes   Rx + Metronidazole
- **Post-influenza**
  - *Staph. aureus*   Rx + Flucloxacillin

Severity score for pneumonia: CURB (2/4)

- Confusion.
- Urea >7.
- Respiratory rate >30.
- **BP** systolic <90 mmHg or diastolic <60 mmHg.

Others: WCC <4 or >12, $T°C$ >38 or <32, age >65, Pao_2 <8, multiple lobes affected.

Severe CAP should receive high-dose IV antibiotics initially.

Prevention

Pneumovax II® to high-risk groups, e.g. chronic disease (especially nephrotic and asplenic patients) and the elderly.

Complications

- Lung abscess (*Staph. aureus*, *Klebsiella*, anaerobes).
- Para-pneumonic effusion/empyema.
- Pneumothorax.

- Haemoptysis.
- Septic shock and multi-organ failure.

Other causes of consolidation
- Tumour.
- Pulmonary embolus.
- Vasculitis, e.g. Churg–Strauss.

Cystic fibrosis

Please examine this young man's chest and comment on what you find.

Clinical signs

- Inspection: small stature, **clubbed**, tachypnoeic, sputum pot (purulent++) and halitosis.
- Hyperinflated with reduced chest expansion and rib recession (Harrison's sulci).
- **Coarse crackles** and wheeze (bronchiectatic).

Extra points

- **Examine the precordium: Portex reservoir** under the skin or **Hickman line/scars** for long-term antibiotics.
- **Cor pulmonale:** cyanosis, ankle oedema, RVH, loud P_2.

Discussion
Genetics

- Incidence of $1/2500$ live births.
- Autosomal recessive chromosome 7q.
- Gene encodes CFTR (Cl^- channel).
- Commonest mutation is a deletion $\Delta508$ (70%).

Pathophysiology
Secretions are thickened and block the lumens of various structures:
- Bronchioles $\rightarrow$ bronchiectasis.
- Pancreatic ducts $\rightarrow$ chronic pancreatitis.
- Gut $\rightarrow$ meconium ileus equivalent in adults.
- Seminal vesicles $\rightarrow$ male infertility.

Investigations

- Screened at birth: low immunoreactive trypsin.
- Sweat test: $Na^+ > 60\,mmol/L$ (false +ive in hypothyroidism and Addison's).
- Genetic screening.

Treatment

- **Physiotherapy:** postural drainage and breathing techniques.
- Antibiotics and bronchodilators.
- Pancrease® and other supplements.

- Immunizations.
- Heart and lung transplant (50% survival at 5 yrs).
- Gene therapy is under development.

Prognosis
Median survival is 30 yrs but is rising. Poor prognosis if becomes infected with *Pseudomonas aeruginosa* and/or *cepacia*, which are difficult to treat.

Chronic obstructive airways disease

Please examine this patient's chest; he has a chronic chest condition.

Clinical signs
- Inspection: nebulizer/inhalers/nasal speculums/sputum pot, dyspnoea, central cyanosis and pursed lips.
- CO_2 retention flap, bounding pulse and tar stained fingers.
- Tracheal tug/accessory muscles ++.
- Hyper-expanded.
- Percussion note resonant.
- Expiratory wheeze (crackles if consolidation too) and reduced breath sounds.

Extra points
- Cor pulmonale: raised JVP, ankle oedema, RV heave and loud P_2.
- COPD does not cause clubbing: therefore, if present consider bronchial carcinoma or bronchiectasis.

Discussion
- Chronic bronchitis: **clinical diagnosis** cough productive of sputum on most days for >3/12 on >2 consecutive years.
- Emphysema: **pathological diagnosis** destruction of alveolar walls.
- Degree of overlap with chronic asthma (main differential diagnosis), although in COPD there tends to be less reversibility (<15%).

Causes
- Environmental: smoking and industrial dust exposure.
- Genetic: α_1-antitrypsin deficiency.

Investigations
- **CXR**: hyper-expanded and/or pneumothorax.
- **ABG**: Type II respiratory failure (low Pao_2 high $Paco_2$).
- **Bloods**: high WCC (infection), low α_1- antitrypsin (younger patients/FH+), low albumin (severity).
- **Spirometry**: low FEV_1 (<40% predicted is severe), $FEV_1/FVC < 0.7$ (obstructive).
- **Gas transfer**: low T_LCO.

Treatment
- **Medical**
  - Bronchodilators.

- Steroid responsiveness trial → symptomatic improvement (10%) then inhaled steroids.
- Aminophylline.
- **Smoking cessation** is the single most beneficial management strategy.
  - Cessation clinics.
  - Pharmacological agents: nicotine replacement and Bupropion.
- **Long-term oxygen therapy (LTOT).**
- Exercise.
- Nutrition (often malnourished).
- Vaccinations.
- **Pulmonary rehabilitation.**
- **Surgical** (careful patient selection is important).
- Bullectomy (if bullae >1 L and compresses surrounding lung).
- Lung reduction surgery.
- Lung transplant.

LTOT
- **Inclusion criteria**
  - Non-smoker.
  - $FEV_1 < 1.5\,L$, $FVC < 2\,L$.
  - $Pao_2 < 7.3\,kPa$ on air.
  - $Paco_2$ that does not rise excessively on O_2.
  - Evidence of cor pulmonale.
- 2–4 L/min via nasal prongs for at least 15 h a day is effective.
- Improves average survival by 9 months.

Treatment of an acute exacerbation
- Controlled O_2 via Venturi mask (24%), monitored closely.
- Bronchodilators.
- Antibiotics.
- Steroids 7–14 days.
- IV Aminophylline.

If acute respiratory failure (↑ $Paco_2$, ↓ Po_2, ↓ pH, ↓ RR and drowsy)
- NIPPV: BIPAP via a face mask.
- IPPV (if first episode of respiratory failure, remediable cause of deterioration and good premorbid quality of life with a reasonable level of activity).

Prognosis
COPD patients have 15% in-hospital mortality.

Lung cancer

Please examine this patient who has had a 3-month history of chronic cough, malaise and weight loss.

Clinical signs

- Cachectic.
- Clubbing and tar-stained fingers.
- Lymphadenopthy: cervical and axillary.
- Tracheal deviation: towards (collapse) or away (effusion) from the lesion.
- Reduced expansion.
- Percussion note dull (collapse/consolidation) or stony dull (effusion).
- Auscultation:
  - Crackles and bronchial breathing (consolidation/collapse).
  - Reduced breath sounds and vocal resonance (effusion).

Extra points

- **Hepatomegaly or bony tenderness**: metastasis.
- **Treatment**
  - Lobectomy scar.
  - **Radiotherapy:** square burn, **tattoo.**
- **Complications:**
  - **Superior vena cava obstruction:** suffused and oedematous face and upper limbs, dilated superficial chest veins and stridor.
  - **Recurrent laryngeal nerve palsy:** hoarse with a 'bovine' cough.
  - **Horner's sign and wasted small muscles of the hand (T1):** Pancoast's tumour.
  - **Endocrine:** gynaecomastia (ectopic βHCG).
  - **Neurological:** Lambert–Eaton myasthenia syndrome, peripheral neuropathy, proximal myopathy and paraneoplastic cerebellar degeneration.
  - **Dermatological:** dermatomyositis (heliotrope rash on eye lids and purple papules on knuckles (Gottron's papules) associated with a raised CK) and acanthosis nigricans.

Discussion

- Commonest malignancy in the Western world.

Types

- Squamous 35%, Small (Oat) 24%, Adeno 21%, Large 19% and Alveolar 1%.

Causes
• **S**moking, **S**carring, **S**oot (asbestos dust) and **S**mog (air pollution).

Management
Investigation order
1 Diagnosis of a mass
   • **CXR:** collapse, mass and hilar lymphadenopathy.
   • **Spiral CT** (so small tumours are not lost between slices during a breath).
2 Determine cell type
   • **Induced sputum cytology**
   • **Biopsy** by **bronchoscopy** (central lesion and collapse) or **percutaneous needle** (peripheral lesion).
3 Stage (**CT/bronchoscopy/mediastinoscopy/thoracoscopy**)
   • **Non-small cell carcinoma (NSCLC): TNM staging to assess operability.**
   • Small cell carcinoma (SCLC): limited or extensive disease.
4 Lung function tests for operability assessment
   • Pneumonectomy contraindicated if $FEV_1 < 1.2\,L$
5 Complications of the tumour
   • Metastasis: ↑ LFTs, ↑ Ca^{++}, ↓ Hb.
   • NSCLC: ↑ PTHrP →↑ Ca^{++}.
   • SCLC: ↑ ACTH, SIADH → Na^+ ↓.

Treatment
• **NSCLC**
   • **Surgery:** lobectomy or pneumonectomy.
   • **Radiotherapy:** single fractionation (weekly) versus hyperfractionation (daily for 10 days).
   • **Chemotherapy:** benefit unknown.
• **SCLC**
   • **Chemotherapy:** benefit with six courses.
Multidisciplinary approach.

Palliative care
• Dexamethasone and radiotherapy for brain metastasis and SVCO.
• Radiotherapy for haemoptysis, bone pain and cough.
• Chemical pleurodesis for effusion.
• Opiates for cough and pain.

Prognosis

		Untreated	Treated
• **SCLC** (median survival)	Limited	3/12	14/12
	Extensive	6/52	10/12
• **NSCLC**	T1N0M0		60/12
	TnN2M0		15/12

Causes of finger clubbing, 'don't *LIGHT up!*'

- **Lung**: **bronchial carcinoma**, suppurative lung disease and cryptogenic fibrosing alveolitis.
- **Inherited** (rare).
- **Gastrointestinal**: inflammatory bowel disease and cirrhosis/hepato-cellular carcinoma.
- **Heart**: infective endocarditis and cyanotic congenital heart disease.
- **Thyroid**: Grave's disease (acropachy).

Skin, Musculoskeletal, Eyes and Endocrine

Psoriasis

Examine this gentleman's skin and discuss the therapeutic options.

Clinical signs
Chronic plaque (classical) type
- Multiple, well-demarcated plaques with a 'salmon-pink', scaly surface.
- Predilection for extensor surfaces.
- Nail involvement:
  - Pitting.
  - Onycholysis.
  - Hyperkeratosis.
  - Discoloration.
- Also check behind ears, scalp and umbilicus.

Extra points
- Koebner phenomenon: plaques at sites of trauma.
- Joint involvement.
- Skin staining from treatment (see below).
- Other types of psoriasis
  - Guttate: multiple 'drop-like' lesions on trunk and limbs.
  - Flexural (not scaly).
  - Palmo-plantar pustular psoriasis.

Discussion
Definition
Epidermal hyperproliferation and accumulation of inflammatory cells.

Treatment
Topical (in- or outpatient)
- **Emollients**
  - Controls scale.
- **Calcipotriol**
  - Vitamin D analogue.
  - Safe, odourless and does not stain.
- **Coal tar**
  - Smelly, inconvenient (long contact time) and occasionally irritant.
  - Stains brown.
- **Dithranol**
  - Stains purple and burns normal skin.
  - Usually effective.
- **Hydrocortisone**

Systemic
- **Cytotoxics**
  - Methotrexate and ciclosporin.
  - Highly effective, but have side-effects.
- **Retinoids**
  - Acitretin.
  - Safe, but teratogenic.

Phototherapy
- UVB.
- Psoralen + UVA (PUVA).

Complications
- **Psoriatic arthropathy** (10%)

Five forms:
- DIP involvement (similar to OA).
- Large joint mono/oligoarthritis.
- Seronegative (similar to RA).
- Sacroilitis (similar to ankylosing spondylitis).
- Arthritis mutilans.
- **Erythroderma**

Guttate psoriasis
- Associated with streptococcal throat infection.
- Resolves in 3 months.

Causes of nail pitting
- **Psoriasis.**
- Lichen planus.
- Alopecia areata.
- Fungal infections.

Koebner phenomenon seen with
- **Psoriasis.**
- Lichen planus.
- Viral warts.
- Vitiligo.
- Sarcoid.

Eczema

Examine this lady's skin and discuss your treatment options.

Clinical signs
Chronic:
- Erythematous, lichenified patches of skin.
- Predominantly flexural.
- Fissures (painful), especially hands and feet.
- Excoriations.
- Secondary bacterial infection.

Extra points
Differential diagnosis
- **Exogenous**
  - Primary irritant dermatitis: may just affect hands.
- **Endogenous**
  - Atopic (see above).
  - Discoid: well-demarcated patches on the trunk and limbs.
  - Pompholyx: bullae on palms and soles.
  - Seborrhoeic dermatitis.

Discussion
Investigations
- History of atopy, e.g. asthma, hay fever and allergy.
- Patch testing.

Treatment
- Avoid precipitants.
- Emollients.
- Topical steroids.
- Anti-histamines for pruritis.
- Antibiotics for secondary infection.
- UV light therapy.

Leg ulcers

Examine this gentleman's legs.

Clinical signs
Venous
- Painless.
- Gaiter area of lower leg.
- **Stigmata of venous hypertension**
  - Varicose veins or scars from vein stripping.
  - Oedema.
  - Lipodermatosclerosis.
  - Varicose eczema.
  - Atrophie blanche.

Arterial
- Painful.
- Distal extremities and pressure points.
- Trophic changes: hairless and paper thin shiny skin.
- Cold with poor capillary refill.
- **Absent distal pulses**.

Neuropathic
- Painless.
- Pressure areas, e.g. under the metatarsal heads.
- **Peripheral neuropathy.**

Extra points
Cause
- **Venous:** look for an abdominal/pelvic mass.
- **Arterial:** check for atrial fibrillation or cardiac murmur.
- **Neuropathic:** look for diabetic signs, Charcot's joint.

Complications
- **Infection:** temperature, pus and cellulites.
- **Malignant change:** Marjolin's ulcer.

Discussion
Other causes
- Vasculitic, e.g. rheumatoid arthritis.
- Neoplastic, e.g. squamous cell carcinoma.

- Infectious, e.g. syphilis.
- Haematological, e.g. sickle cell anaemia.
- Tropical, e.g. cutaneous leishmaniasis.

Investigations
Venous
- Doppler ultrasound of venous system.

Arterial
- Ankle-Brachial Pressure Index (0.8–1.2 is normal, <0.8 implies arterial insufficiency).
- Arteriography.

NB. Many patients have contact dermatitis to previous topical treatments and dressings.

Treatment
Venous
- Remove exudate and slough with regular cleaning.
- Treat surrounding venous eczema.
- Four-layer compression bandaging.
- Vein surgery.

Arterial
- Angioplasty.
- Vascular reconstruction.
- Amputation.

Causes of neuropathic ulcers
- Diabetes mellitus.
- Tabes dorsalis.
- Syringomyelia.

Diabetes and the skin

This 32-year-old female has Type 1 diabetes mellitus. Please examine her skin.

Clinical signs
Hands
- **Cheiroarthropathy**
  - Tight waxy skin that limits finger extension ('Prayer sign').
- **Granuloma annulare** (10% associated with type 1 diabetes)
  - Flesh-coloured papules in annular configurations on the dorsum of the fingers (and feet).

Shins
- **Necrobiosis lipoidica diabeticorum**
  - Well-demarcated plaques with waxy-yellow centre and red–brown edges.
  - Prominent skin blood vessels.
- **Diabetic dermopathy**
  - Common red/brown, atrophic lesions.

Feet and legs
- **Ulcers:** arterial or neuropathic (see leg ulcer section).
- **Eruptive xanthomata**
  - Yellow papules on buttocks and knees (also elbows).
  - Caused by hyperlipidaemia.

Injection sites
- **Lipoatrophy.**
- **Fat hypertrophy.**

Cutaneous infections
- **Cellulitis.**
- **Candidiasis (intertrigo).**

Extra points
- **Vitiligo** (associated auto-immune disease).
- **Other diabetic complications**
e.g. Charcot joints associated with neuropathic ulcers.

Discussion

Treatment for necrobiosis lipoidica diabeticorum

- Topical steroid and support bandaging.
- Tight glycaemic control does not help.

Xanthomata

- **Hypercholesterolaemia:** tendon xanthomata, xanthelasma and corneal arcus.
- **Hypertriglyceridaemia:** eruptive xanthomata and lipaemia retinalis.
- **Other causes of secondary hyperlipidaemia**
  - Hypothyroidism.
  - Nephrotic syndrome.
  - Alcohol.
  - Cholestasis.

Skin malignancy

Examine this lady's skin/a specific lesion or area of skin.

Basal cell carcinoma

Clinical signs
- Usually on face/trunk: sun-exposed areas.
- Pearly nodule with rolled edge.
- Superficial telangiectasia.
- Ulceration in advanced lesions.

Extra points
- Local invasion and distant metastasis (lymph nodes or hepatomegaly).
- Other lesions.

Discussion
Natural history
- Slowly grow over a few months.
- Local invasion only, rarely metastasize.

Treatment
- Curettage/cryotherapy if superficial.
- Surgical excision +/− radiotherapy.

Squamous cell carcinoma

Clinical signs
- Sun-exposed areas (+ lips + mouth).
- Actinic keratoses: pre-malignant (red, scaly patches).
- Varied appearance
  - Keratotic nodule.
  - Polypoid mass.
  - Cutaneous ulcer.

Extra points
- Local invasion and distant metastasis (lymph nodes or hepatomegaly).
- Other lesions.

Discussion
Diagnosis
- Biopsy suspicious lesions.

Treatment
- Surgery $+/-$ radiotherapy.
- 5% metastasize.

Malignant melanoma

Clinical signs
- Patient's appearance: mention risks
  - Fair skin with freckles.
  - Light hair.
  - Blue eyes.
- Appearance of lesion

Asymmetrical.

Border irregularity.

Colour (black—often irregular pigmentation).

Diameter >6 mm.

Extra points
- Local invasion and distant metastasis (lymph nodes and/or hepato-megaly).
- Other lesions.

Discussion

Diagnosis/treatment
- Excision.
- Staged on Breslow thickness (maximal depth of tumour invasion into dermis):
  - <1.5 mm = 90% 5-yr survival, >3.5 mm = 40% 5-yr survival.

Beware the man with a glass eye and ascites: ocular melanoma!

Other skin problems

Examine this patient's skin.

Pseudoxanthoma elasticum

Clinical signs

- 'Plucked chicken skin' appearance: loose skin folds especially at the neck and axillae, with yellow pseudoxanthomatous plaques.
- Hyperextensible joints.

Extra points

Eyes

- Blue sclerae.
- Reduced visual acuity.
- Retinal angioid streaks and macular degeneration.

Cardiovascular

- Blood pressure: 50% are hypertensive.
- Mitral valve prolapse.
- CVA and/or CCF from atherosclerosis.

Discussion

- Inheritance: autosomal dominant or recessive.
- Degenerative elastic fibres in skin, blood vessels and eye.
- Premature coronary artery disease.

Ehlers–Danlos

Clinical signs

- Early scarring: 'fish-mouth' scars especially on the knees. No skin folds.
- Fragile skin: multiple ecchymoses.
- Hyperextensible skin: able to tent up skin when pulled (avoid doing this).
- Joint hypermobility and dislocation.

Extra points

- Mitral valve prolapse.
- Abdominal scars
  - Aneurysmal rupture and dissection.
  - Bowel perforation and bleeding.

Discussion
- Inheritance: autosomal dominant.
- Defect in collagen causing increased skin elasticity.
- No premature coronary artery disease.

Osler–Weber–Rendu (hereditary haemorrhagic telangiectasia)

Clinical signs
- Multiple telangiectasia on the face, lips and buccal mucosa.

Extra points
- Anaemia: gastrointestinal bleeding.
- Cyanosis and chest bruit: pulmonary vascular abnormality/shunt.

Discussion
- Autosomal dominant.
- Increased risk gastrointestinal haemorrhage, epistaxis, and haemoptysis.
- Vascular malformations:
  - Pulmonary shunts.
  - Intracranial aneurysms: subarachnoid haemorrhage.

Erythema nodosum

Clinical signs
- Tender, red nodules commonly found on the shins.
- Older lesions leave a bruise.

Extra points
- Signs of a cause, e.g. red, sore throat or systemic manifestations of sarcoidosis.

Discussion
- Pathology: inflammation of subcutaneous fat (panniculitis).
- Associations
  - **Streptococcal infections.**
  - **Sarcoidosis.**
  - **Streptomycin.**
  - Also TB, IBD and lymphoma.
- Other skin manifestations of sarcoidosis
  - **Nodules and papules:** red/brown seen particularly around the face, nose, ears and neck. Demonstrates Koebner's phenomenon.
  - **Lupus pernio:** diffuse bluish/brown plaque with central small papules commonly affecting the nose.

Tuberous sclerosis

Please examine this lady's skin. What is the diagnosis?

Clinical signs
- Facial (perinasal) adenoma sebaceum (angiofibromata).
- Periungual fibromas (hands and feet).
- Shagreen patch: roughened skin over the lumbar region.
- Ash leaf macules: depigmented areas on trunk (fluoresce with UV/ Wood's light).

Extra points
Respiratory
- Cystic lung disease.

Abdominal
- Polycystic kidneys.
- Transplanted kidney.
- Dialysis fistulae.

Eyes
- Retinal phakomas (dense white patches) in 50%.

CNS
- Mental retardation.

Signs of anti-epileptic treatment, e.g. phenytoin: gum hypertrophy and hirsutism.

Discussion
- Autosomal dominant.
- 80% epileptic.

Investigation
- Skull films: 'Railroad track' calcification.
- CT/MRI head: tuberous masses in cerebral cortex. Often calcify.

Also known as **EPILOIA**

EPIlepsy

LOw Intelligence

Adenoma sebaceum

Neurofibromatosis

Examine this patient's skin.

Clinical signs
- Cutaneous neurofibromas.
- Café au Lait patches: five or more.
- Axillary freckling.
- Lisch nodules: melanocytic hamartomas of the iris.

Extra points
- Blood pressure: hypertension (associated with renal artery stenosis and phaeochromocytoma).
- Examine the chest: fine crackles (honeycomb lung and fibrosis).
- Neuropathy with enlarged palpable nerves.

Discussion
- Inheritance is autosomal dominant.
- Type I is the classical peripheral form, type II is central and presents with bilateral acoustic neuromas and sensi-neural deafness rather than skin lesions.

Associations
- Phaeochromocytoma (2%).
- Renal artery stenosis (2%).

Complications
- Epilepsy.
- Sarcomatous change (5%).
- Scoliosis (5%).
- Mental retardation (10%).

Causes of enlarged nerves and peripheral neuropathy
- **Neurofibromatosis.**
- Leprosy.
- Amyloidosis.
- Acromegaly.
- Refsum's disease.

Rheumatoid arthritis

Examine this lady's hands.

Clinical signs
- Symmetrical, deforming polyarthropathy.
- Volar subluxation and ulnar deviation at the MCPJs.
- Subluxation at the wrist.
- Swan-neck deformity (hyperextension of the PIPJ and flexion of the DIPJ).
- Boutonnière's deformity (flexion of the PIPJ and hyperextension of the DIPJ).
- 'Z' thumbs.
- Rheumatoid nodules (elbows).
- Muscle wasting (disuse atrophy).

Assess disease activity
- Red, swollen, hot, painful hands imply active disease.

Assess function
- **Power grip:** 'Squeeze my fingers'.
- **Precision grip:** 'Pick up a coin' or 'Do up your buttons'.
- **Key grip:** 'Pretend to use this key'.
- Remember the wheelchair, walking aids and splints.

Extra points
- Exclude psoriatic arthropathy (main differential):
  - Nail changes.
  - Psoriasis: elbows, behind ears, scalp and around the umbilicus.
- Surgical scars:
  - Carpal tunnel release (wrist).
  - Joint replacement (especially thumb).
  - Tendon transfer (dorsum of hand).
- Steroid side effects.
- C-spine stabilization scars.
- Systemic manifestations (see below).

Discussion
Systemic manifestations of RA
- **Pulmonary:**
  - Pleural effusions.
  - Fibrosing alveolitis.

- Obliterative bronchiolitis.
- Caplan's nodules.
- **Eyes**:
  - Dry (Secondary Sjögren's).
  - Scleritis.
- **Neurological**:
  - Carpal tunnel syndrome (commonest).
  - Atlanto-axial subluxation: quadriplegia.
  - Peripheral neuropathy.
- **Haematological**:
  - Felty's syndrome: RA + splenomegaly + neutropenia.
  - Anaemia (all types!).
- **Cardiac:**
  - Pericarditis.

Investigations
- Elevated inflammatory markers.
- Radiological changes:
  - Soft tissue swelling.
  - Loss of joint space.
  - Articular erosions.
  - Periarticular osteoporosis.
- Positive rheumatoid factor in 80%.

Diagnosis– 4/7 of American College of Rheumatology criteria
- Morning stiffness.
- Arthritis in 3+ joint areas.
- Arthritis of hands.
- Symmetrical arthritis.
- Rheumatoid nodules.
- Positive rheumatoid factor.
- Erosions on joint radiographs.

Treatment
- Explanation and education.
- Exercise and physiotherapy.
- Occupational therapy and social support.
- Symptomatic relief: NSAIDs and COX-2 inhibitors.
- Disease-modifying anti-rheumatic drugs:

	Serious side effects	Monitor
• Hydroxychloroquine	Retinopathy	Visual acuity
• Sulphasalazine	Rash and bone marrow suppression	FBC
• Corticosteroids	Osteoporosis	
• Azathioprine	Neutropenia	FBC
• Methotrexate	Neutropenia, pulmonary toxicity, hepatitis	CXR, FBC, LFT
• Gold complexes	Thrombocytopenia, rash	FBC
• Penicillamine	Proteinuria, thrombocytopenia rash	FBC and urine
• Infliximab/Etanercept	Rash, immunosuppression	

• Surgery (joint replacement, tendon transfer, etc.)

Systemic lupus erythematosus

Please examine this lady's skin and discuss your findings.

Clinical signs
Face
- Malar 'butterfly' rash.
- Photosensitivity.
- Discoid rash +/− scarring (Discoid Lupus).
- Oral ulceration.
- Scarring alopecia.
- Anaemia.

Hands
- Vasculitic lesions (nail-fold infarcts).
- Raynaud's phenomenon.
- Jaccoud's arthropathy (mimics rheumatoid arthritis but due to tendon contractures not joint destruction).

Elsewhere
- Livedo reticularis.
- Purpura.
- Peripheral oedema (nephrotic syndrome).

Extra points
- Respiratory:
  - Pleural effusion.
  - Pleural rub.
  - Fibrosing alveolitis.
- Neurological:
  - Focal neurology.
  - Chorea.
  - Ataxia.
- Eyes:
  - Dry (Sjögren's).
Reno-vascular:
  - Hypertension.
  - Proteinuria.

Discussion
Diagnostic investigation
- Serum autoantibodies (ANA, **anti-dsDNA**).

Disease activity
- Elevated ESR but normal CRP (raised CRP too indicates infection).
- Elevated immunoglobulins.
- Reduced complement (C_4).
- U+Es, urine microscopy (glomerulonephritis).

Diagnosis—4/11 of American College of Rheumatology criteria
- Malar rash.
- Discoid rash.
- Photosensitivity.
- Oral ulcers.
- Arthritis.
- Serositis (pleuritis or pericarditis).
- Renal involvement (proteinuria or cellular casts).
- Neurological disorder (seizures or psychosis).
- Haematological disorder (autoimmune haemolytic anaemia or pancytopenia).
- Immunological disorders (positive anti-dsDNA or anti-Sm antibodies).
- Elevated titre of anti-nuclear antibody (ANA).

Treatment
- **Mild disease (cutaneous/joint involvement only):**
  - Topical corticosteroids.
  - Hydroxychloroquine.
- **Moderate disease (+ other organ involvement):**
  - Prednisolone.
  - Azathioprine.
- **Severe disease (+ severe inflammatory involvement of vital organs):**
  - Methylprednisolone.
  - Cyclophosphamide.
  - Azathioprine.

Cyclophosphamide side-effects
- Haematological and Haemorrhagic cystitis.
- Infertility.
- Teratogenicity.

Prognosis
- Good: 90% survival at 10 yrs.

Systemic sclerosis

Please examine this lady's skin.

Clinical signs
Hands
- Sclerodactyly.
- Calcinosis (may ulcerate).
- Raynaud's **phenomenon** (Raynaud's disease is idiopathic!).

Face
- Tight skin.
- Beaked nose.
- Microstomia.
- Peri-oral furrowing.
- Telangiectasia.
- Alopecia.

Other skin lesions
- Morphoea: focal/generalized patches of sclerotic skin.
- En coup de sabre (scar down central forehead).
Attempt to classify the disease (see below).

Extra points
- **Blood pressure:**
  - Hypertension.
- **Respiratory:**
  - Interstitial fibrosis (fine, bibasal crackles).
- **Cardiac:**
  - Pulmonary hypertension (RV heave, loud P_2 and TR).
  - Evidence of failure.
  - Pericarditis (rub).
- Raynaud's (colour change order: white (vasoconstriction) $\rightarrow$ blue (cyanosis) $\rightarrow$ red (hyperaemia)).

Discussion
Classification
- **Localized:** morphea to patch of skin only.
- **Systemic: limited** and **diffuse.**

Limited systemic sclerosis
- Distribution limited to hands, feet and face
- Slow progression (years)
- Includes **CREST**:
  Calcinosis
  Raynaud's phenomenon
  oEsophageal dysmotility
  Sclerodactyly
  Telangiectasia

Diffuse systemic sclerosis
- Widespread cutaneous and early visceral involvement
- Rapid progression (months)

Investigations
- **Autoantibodies:**
  - Anti-nuclear antibody positive (in 90%).
  - Anti-centromere antibody = Limited (in 80%).
  - Scl-70 antibody = Diffuse (in 70%).
- **Hand radiographs:** calcinosis.
- **Pulmonary disease: lower lobe fibrosis and aspiration pneumonia**
  - CXR, high resolution CT scan and pulmonary function tests.
- **Gastrointestinal disease: dysmotility and malabsorption**
  - Contrast scans, FBC and B12/folate.
- **Renal disease: glomerulonephritis**
  - U+E, urinalysis, urine microscopy (casts) and consider renal biopsy.
- **Cardiac disease: myocardial fibrosis and arrhythmias**
  - ECG and ECHO.

Treatment
Symptomatic treatment only:
- Camouflage creams.
- **Raynaud's therapy:**
  - Gloves, hand-warmers, etc.
  - Calcium channel blockers.
  - ACE inhibitors.
  - Prostacyclin infusion (severe).
- **Renal:**
  - ACE inhibitors: prevent hypertensive crisis and reduce the mortality from renal failure.
- **Gastrointestinal:**
  - Proton-pump inhibitor for oesophageal reflux.

Prognosis
Mean 5-yr survival of diffuse systemic sclerosis is 50%. Most deaths are due to respiratory failure.

Ankylosing spondylitis

Examine this patient's posture and then proceed to demonstrate any other features of this disease.

Clinical signs
- Question mark posture caused by fixed kyphoscoliosis and loss of lumbar lordosis with extension of cervical spine.
- Reduced range of movement throughout entire spine.
- Protuberant abdomen due to diaphragmatic breathing.
- Reduced chest expansion (<5 cm increase in girth).
- Increased Occiput – Wall distance (>5 cm).
- **Schöber's Test:** Two points marked 15 cm apart on the dorsal spine expand by less than 5 cm on maximum forward flexion.

Extra points
Complications you should look for:
- Anterior Uveitis (commonest 30%).
- Apical lung fibrosis.
- Aortic regurgitation (4%).
- Atrio-ventricular nodal heart block (10%).
- Arthritis.

Remember psoriatic arthropathy may present in a very similar way so look for plaques.

Discussion
Genetics
- 90% association with HLA B27.

Treatment
- Physiotherapy.
- Analgesia.

Marfan's syndrome

> *Examine this man's hands and then proceed to examine anything else that will help you make a diagnosis.*

Clinical signs
General (spot diagnosis)
• **Tall** with **long extremities** (arm span > height).

Hands
• **Arachnodactyly**: can encircle their wrist with thumb and little finger.
• **Hyperextensible joints**: thumb able to touch ipsilateral wrist and adduct over the palm with its tip visible at the ulnar boarder.

Face
• **High arched palate** with crowded teeth.
• Iridodonesis (with upward lens dislocation).

Chest
• Pectus carinatum ('pigeon') or excavatum.
• Scoliosis.
• Scars from cardiac surgery.

Extra points
Cardiac
• Aortic incompetence: collapsing pulse.
• Mitral valve prolapse.
• Coarctation.

Chest
• Pneumothorax: scars from chest drains.

Abdominal
• Inguinal herniae and scars.

CNS
• Normal IQ.

Discussion
Genetics
• Autosomal dominant, chromosome 15.

- Defect in fibrillin protein (connective tissue).

Management
- **Surveillance:** monitoring of aortic root size with annual trans-thoracic echo.
- **Treatment:** β-blockers to slow aortic root dilatation and preemptive aortic root surgery to prevent dissection and aortic rupture.
- **Screen family members.**

Differential diagnosis
- Homocystinuria
  - Mental retardation and downward lens dislocation.

Paget's disease

Examine this gentleman and discuss his diagnosis.

Clinical signs
- Bony enlargement: skull and long bones (sabre tibia).
- Deafness (conductive): hearing-aid.
- Pathological fractures: scars.

Extra points
- Cardiac failure (high-output): elevated JVP, ankle oedema, dyspnoea.
- Entrapment neuropathies: carpal tunnel syndrome.
- Optic atrophy and angioid streaks.

Discussion
Symptoms
- Usually asymptomatic.
- Bone pain and tenderness (2%).

Investigations
- Grossly elevated alkaline phosphatase, normal calcium and phosphate.
- Radiology:
  - 'Moth-eaten' appearance on plain films: osteoporosis circumscripta.
  - Bone scans (↑ uptake).

Treatment
- Symptomatic: analgesia, hearing aid.
- Bisphosphonates.

Other complications
- Osteogenic sarcoma (1%).
- Basilar invagination (cord compression).
- Kidney stones.

Causes of sabre tibia
- **Paget's.**
- Osteomalacia.
- Syphilis.

Causes of angioid streaks
- **Paget's.**
- Pseudoxanthoma elasticum.
- Ehlers–Danlos.

Other joint problems

Examine this man's hands.

Tophaceous gout

Clinical signs
- Asymmetrical swelling of the small joints of the hands and feet (commonly first MTPJ).
- Gouty tophi (chalky white deposits) seen around the joints, ear and tendons.
- Reduced movement and function.

Extra points
- **Associations:**
  - Obesity.
  - Hypertension.
  - Urate stones/nephropathy: nephrectomy scars.
- **Cause:**
  - Drug card: diuretics.
  - Lymphadenopathy: lymphoproliferative disorder.
  - Chronic renal failure: fistulae.

Discussion
Cause
- Urate excess.

Investigation
- Uric acid levels (unreliable).
- Synovial fluid: needle-shaped, negatively birefringent crystals.
- Radiograph features: 'punched out' periarticular changes.

Treatment
- **Acute attack:**
  - Treat the cause.
  - Increase hydration.
  - High dose NSAIDs.
  - Colchicine and high fluid intake.
- **Prevention**
  - Avoid precipitants.
  - Allopurinol (xanthine oxidase inhibitor).

Osteoarthritis

Clinical signs
- Elderly patient ± walking stick.
- Asymmetrical distal interphalangeal joint deformity with Heberden's nodes (and sometimes Bouchard's nodes at the proximal interphalangeal joint).
- Disuse atrophy of hand muscles.
- Crepitation, reduced movement and function.

Extra points
- Carpal tunnel syndrome or scars.
- Other joint involvement and joint replacement scars.

Discussion
Prevalence: 20% (common).

Radiographic features
- Loss of joint space.
- Osteophytes.
- Peri-articular sclerosis and cysts.

Treatment
- Simple analgesia.
- Weight reduction (if OA affects weight bearing joint).
- Physiotherapy and occupational therapy.
- Joint replacement.

Diabetic retinopathy

This patient has had difficulty with his/her vision. Please examine his/her eyes.

Clinical signs
- Look around for clues—a white stick, braille book or glucometer.
- Fundoscopy: check for red reflex (absent if cataract or vitreous haemorrhage).

Tip: find the disc (inferonasally) then follow each of the four main vessels out to the periphery of the quadrants and finish by examining the macular 'look at the light'.

Extra points
- Check for coexisting hypertensive changes (they always ask!).

Discussion
Screening
- <40 yrs old: every 2 yrs.
- >40 yrs old or more than 10 yrs since diagnosis: annual.

Test acuity, fundoscopy and retinal photography/fluoroscein angiography.
- Background retinopathy usually occurs 10–20 yrs after diabetes is diagnosed.
- Young type I diabetics often get proliferative retinopathy whereas older type II diabetics tend to get exudative maculopathy.

Treatment
Tight glycaemic control
- Lower blood sugar (HbA_{1c} <7.5%) is associated with less retinopathy.
- There may be a transient worsening of the retinopathy initially.

Treat hypertension and hypercholesterolaemia
- BP <140/80 improves micro- and macrovascular complication rates (UKPDS).

Photocoagulation
Indications
- Maculopathy.
- Proliferative and preproliferative diabetic retinopathy.

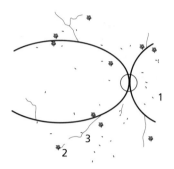

Background retinopathy

1 Hard exudates
2 Blot haemorrhages
3 Microaneurysms

Routine referral to eye clinic.

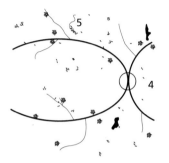

Pre-proliferative retinopathy

Background changes plus
4 Cotton wool spots
5 Flame haemorrhages
Also venous beading and loops and IRMAs (intraretinal microvascular abnormalities).

Urgent referral to ophthalmology.

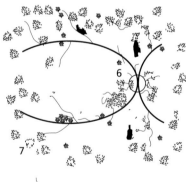

Proliferative retinopathy

Pre-proliferative changes plus
6 Neovascularization of the disc (NVD) and elsewhere
7 Panretinal photocoagulation scars (treatment)

Urgent referral to ophthalmology.

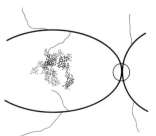

Diabetic maculopathy

Macular oedema or hard exudates within one disc space of the fovea.

Treated with focal photocoagulation.

Urgent referral to ophthalmology.

Pan-retinal photocoagulation prevents the ischaemic retinal cells secreting angiogenesis factors causing neovascularization. Focal photocoagulation targets problem vessels at risk of bleeding.

Accelerated deterioration occurs in poor diabetic control, hypertension and pregnancy.

Hypertensive retinopathy

Examine this patient's fundus.

Clinical signs

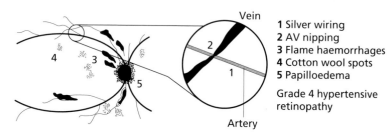

Vein

1 Silver wiring
2 AV nipping
3 Flame haemorrhages
4 Cotton wool spots
5 Papilloedema

Grade 4 hypertensive
retinopathy

Artery

Grade 1: silver wiring (increased reflectance from thickened arterioles).
Grade 2: plus AV nipping (narrowing of veins as arterioles cross them).
Grade 3: plus cotton wool spots and flame haemorrhages.
Grade 4: plus papilloedema.
There may also be hard exudates (macular star).

Extra points
Causes
- Essential 94%.
- Renal 4%: renal bruit or enlarged kidneys.
- Endocrine 1%: acromegaly, Cushing's or phaeochromocytoma.
- Coarctation: radio-femoral delay.
- Eclampsia: pregnancy.

Common causes of papilloedema
- Raised intracranial pressure: space occupying lesion, benign intracranial hypertension and cavernous sinus thrombosis.
- Malignant hypertension.
- Central retinal vein occlusion.

Papilloedema: normal visual acuity, obscurations and tunnel vision.
Papillitis: reduced visual acuity and central scotoma.

Discussion
Malignant hypertension
- Medical emergency.

Treatment
- Grade III and IV retinopathy and hypertension.

Oral anti-hypertensives.
- Plus encephalopathy/stroke/myocardial infarction/left ventricular failure.

Parenteral venodilators.

Over-rapid fall in blood pressure can lead to cerebral and retinal infarction.

Retinitis pigmentosa

This man has been complaining of difficulty seeing at night. Please examine his eyes.

Clinical signs
- White stick and braille book (registered blind).
- Reduced peripheral field of vision (tunnel vision).
- Fundoscopy

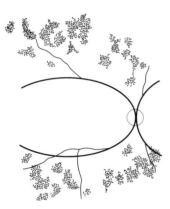

Peripheral retina 'bone spicule pigmentation', which follows the veins and spares the macula.

Optic atrophy due to neuronal loss (consecutive).

Association: cataract (absent red reflex).

Extra points
'At a glance' findings can help make the diagnosis
- **Ataxic:** Friedreich's ataxia, abetalipoproteinaemia, Refsum's disease, Kearns–Sayre syndrome.
- **Deafness (hearing-aid/white stick with red stripes):** Refsum's disease, Kearns–Sayre syndrome, Usher's disease.
- **Ophthalmoplegia/ptosis and permanent pacemaker:** Kearns–Sayre syndrome.
- **Polydactyly:** Laurence–Moon–Biedl syndrome.
- **Icthyosis:** Refsum's disease.

Discussion
Causes
- Congenital: see above (often autosomal recessive inheritance).
- Acquired: post-inflammatory retinitis.

Prognosis

- Progressive loss of vision due to retinal degeneration. Most are registered blind at 40 yrs, with central visual loss in the seventh decade.
- No treatment.

Causes of tunnel vision

- Papilloedema.
- Glaucoma.
- Choroidoretinitis.
- Migraine.
- Hysteria.

Retinal artery occlusion

Examine this gentleman's fundi

Clinical signs
• Pale, milky fundus with thread-like arterioles.
• ± Cherry red macula (choroidal blood supply).

Extra points
• **Cause:** AF (irregular pulse) or carotid stenosis (bruit).
• **Effect:** optic atrophy and blind (white stick).
NB. Branch retinal artery occlusion will have a field defect opposite to the quadrant of affected retina.

Discussion
Causes
• **Embolic:** carotid plaque rupture or cardiac mural thrombus.
Rx: Aspirin, anti-coagulation and endarterectomy.
• **Giant cell arteritis:** tender scalp and pulseless temporal arteries.
Rx: High dose steroid urgently.

Retinal vein occlusion

Examine this patient's fundi

Clinical signs
- Flame haemorrhages + + + radiating out from a swollen disc.
- Engorged tortuous veins.
- Cotton wool spots.

Extra points
- **Cause:** Look for diabetic or hypertensive changes (visible in branch retinal vein occlusion).
- **Effect:** Rubeosis iridis causes secondary glaucoma (in central retinal vein occlusion), visual loss or field defect.

Discussion
Causes
- **Hypertension.**
- **Hyperglycaemia:** diabetes mellitus.
- **Hyperviscocity:** Waldenström's macroglobulinaemia or myeloma.
- **High intraocular pressure:** glaucoma.

Abnormal pupils

Examine this patient's eyes.

Horner's pupil

Clinical signs

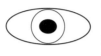

Horner's

'PEAS'
Ptosis (levator palpebrae is
partially supplied by sympathetic
fibres)
Enophthalmos (sunken eye)
Anhydrosis (sympathetic fibres
control sweating)
Small pupil (miosis)

May also have flushed/warm skin
ipsilaterally to the Horner's pupil
due to loss of vasomotor
sympathetic tone to the face.

Extra points

• Look at the ipsilateral side of the neck for scars (trauma, e.g. central lines, carotid endarterectomy surgery or aneurysms) and tumours (Pancoast's).

Discussion
Cause
Following the sympathetic tract's anatomical course:

Brain stem	**Spinal cord**	**Neck**
MS	Syrinx	Aneurysm
Stroke (Wallenberg's)		Trauma
		Pancoast's

Holmes–Adie (myotonic) pupil

Clinical signs

Holmes–Adie pupil

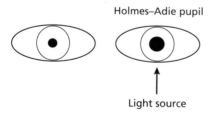

Light source

Moderately dilated pupil that
has a poor response to light
and a sluggish response
to accommodation
(you may have to wait!)

Extra points
• Absent or diminished ankle and knee jerks.

Discussion
A benign condition that is more common in females. Reassure the patient that nothing is wrong.

Argyll Robertson pupil

Clinical signs

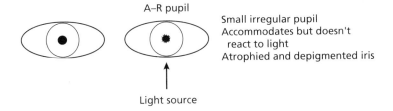

A–R pupil

Small irregular pupil
Accommodates but doesn't
  react to light
Atrophied and depigmented iris

Light source

Extra points
• Offer to look for sensory ataxia (tabes dorsalis).

Discussion
• Usually a manifestation of quaternary syphilis, but it may also be caused by diabetes mellitus.
• Test for quaternary syphilis using TPHA or FTA, which remain positive for the duration of the illness.
• Treat with penicillin.

Oculomotor (III) nerve palsy

Clinical signs

Ptosis usually complete
Dilated pupil
The eye points 'down and out' due
to the unopposed action of lateral
rectus (VI) and superior oblique (IV)

III nerve palsy

Extra points

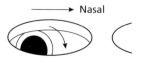

→ Nasal

Test for the trochlear (IV) nerve
On looking nasally the eye will intort (rotate towards the nose) indicating that the trochlear nerve is working

- If the pupil is normal consider medical causes of III palsy.
- Surgical causes often impinge on the superficially located papillary fibres running in the III nerve.

Discussion
Causes

Medical	Surgical
Mononeuritis multiplex, e.g. DM	Communicating artery aneurysm (posterior)
Midbrain infarction: Weber's	Cavernous sinus pathology: thrombosis, tumour or
Midbrain demyelination	fistula (IV, V, VI may also be affected)
Migraine	Cerebral uncus herniation

Optic atrophy

Examine this woman's eyes.

Clinical signs

- Relative afferent papillary defect (RAPD): dilatation of the pupil on moving the light source from the normal eye (consensual reflex) to the abnormal eye (direct reflex):

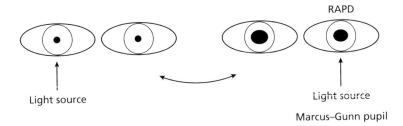

- Fundoscopy: disc pallor.

Extra points

Look for the cause.

On examining the fundus

- **Glaucoma** (cupping of the disc).
- **Retinitis pigmentosa.**
- **Central retinal artery occlusion.**
- **Frontal brain tumour: Foster–Kennedy syndrome** (papilloedema in one eye due to raised intercranial pressure and optic atrophy in the other due to direct compression by the tumour).

At a glance from the end of the bed

- Cerebellar signs, e.g. nystagmus: **multiple sclerosis** (internuclear ophthalmoplegia), **Friedreich's ataxia** (scoliosis, pes cavus).
- Large bossed skull: **Paget's disease** (hearing aid).
- Argyll Robertson pupil: **Tertiary syphilis.**

Discussion

Causes: PALE DISCS (* commonest)

PRESSURE*: tumour, glaucoma, Paget's
ATAXIA: Friedreich's ataxia
LEBER'S

DIETARY: ↓ B_{12}, DEGENERATIVE: retinitis pigmentosa
ISCHAEMIA: central retinal artery occlusion
SYPHILIS and other infections, e.g. CMV, toxoplasmosis
CYANIDE and other toxins, e.g. alcohol, lead, tobacco
SCLEROSIS*: MS

Hyperthyroidism and Graves' disease

This lady presents with a lump in her neck. Please examine it.

Clinical signs
- Smooth, diffuse goitre

	Specific to Graves'	**Hyperthyroidism**
Eye signs	• Proptosis	• Lid retraction
	• Chemosis	• Lid lag
	• Exposure keratitis	
	• Ophthalmoplegia	
Peripheral signs	• Thyroid acropachy	• Agitation
	• Pretibial myxoedema	• Sweating
		• Tremor
		• Palmar erythema
		• Sinus tachycardia/AF
		• Brisk reflexes

Extra points
Thyroid status
- Graves' disease patients may be hyperthyroid, euthyroid or hypothyroid depending on their stage of treatment.

Eyes
- Keratitis is due to poor eye closure.
- Optic nerve compression: loss of colour vision initially then development of a central scotoma and reduced visual acuity.
- Papilloedema may occur.

Discussion
Investigation
- Thyroid function tests: TSH and T_3/T_4.
- Thyroid autoantibodies.
- Radioisotope scanning: increased uptake of I^{131} in Graves', reduced in thyroiditis.

Treatment
- β-blocker, e.g. Propranolol.
- Carbimazole or Propylthiouracil (both thionamides). Either

- **Block and replace** with thyroxine.
- **Titrate** dose and monitor endogenous thyroxine.

Stop at 18 months and assess for return of thyrotoxicosis. One-third of patients will remain euthyroid.

If thyrotoxicosis returns, the options are
- A repeat course of a thionamide.
- Radioiodine (I^{131}): hypothyroidism common.
- Subtotal thyroidectomy.
- Severe ophthalmopathy may require high-dose steroids, orbital irradiation or surgical decompression to prevent visual loss.

The **NOSPECS** mnemonic for the progression of eye signs in Graves':

No signs or symptoms

Only lid lag/retraction

Soft tissue involvement

Proptosis

Extraocular muscle involvement

Chemosis

Sight loss due to optic nerve compression and atrophy

Hypothyroidism

Examine this patient—she has been complaining of the cold.

Clinical signs
- **Hands:**
  - Slow pulse.
  - Dry skin.
  - Cool peripheries.
- **Head/face/neck:**
  - 'Peaches and cream' complexion (anaemia and carotenaemia).
  - Eyes: peri-orbital oedema, loss of eyebrows and xanthelasma.
  - Thinning hair.
  - Goitre or thyroidectomy scar.
- **Legs:**
  - Slow relaxing ankle jerk (tested with patient kneeling on a chair).

Extra points
Complications
- **Cardiac:** pericardial effusion (rub), congestive cardiac failure (oedema).
- **Neurological:** Carpel tunnel syndrome (Phalen's/Tinel's test), proximal myopathy (stand from sitting) and ataxia.

Other autoimmune diseases
- Addison's disease, vitiligo and diabetes mellitus.

Discussion
Investigation
- **Blood:** TSH ($\uparrow$ in thyroid failure, $\downarrow$ in pituitary failure), T_4 $\downarrow$
Autoantibodies
Associations: U+E: Na^+ $\downarrow$, hypercholesterolaemia, FBC: macrocytic anaemia.
- **Urine:** 24-h collection for cortisol (exclude Addison's).
- **ECG:** pericardial effusion and ischaemia.
- **CXR:** pericardial effusion and CCF.

Management
- Thyroxine titrated to TSH suppression and clinical response.
- NB.　1 Can precipitate angina.
　　　2 Can unmask Addison's disease → crisis.

Causes

- **Autoimmune:** Hashimoto's thyroiditis (+goitre) and atrophic hypo-thyroidism.
- **Iatrogenic:** Post-thyroidectomy or I^{131}, amiodarone, lithium and anti-thyroid drugs.
- **Iodine deficiency:** dietary ('Derbyshire neck').
- **Dyshormonogenesis.**

Acromegaly

*Please examine this man who has been complaining of headaches.**

Clinical signs: 'spot diagnosis'
- **Hands:** large 'spade like', **tight rings*,** coarse skin and **sweaty*.**
- **Face:** prominent supra-orbital ridges, prognathism, widely spaced teeth and macroglossia.

(**Signs of active disease.**)

Extra points
Complications to look for: **A, B, C...**
  Acanthosis nigricans
  BP ↑*
  Carpal tunnel syndrome
  Diabetes mellitus*
  Enlarged organs
  Field defect*: bitemporal hemianopia
  Goitre, Gastrointestinal malignancy
  Heart failure, Hirsute, Hypopituitary
  IGF-1 ↑
  Joint arthropathy
  Kyphosis
  Lactation (galactorrhoea)
  Myopathy (proximal)

Discussion
Investigations
Diagnostic
- **Non-suppression of GH** after an oral glucose tolerance test.
- Raised plasma **IGF-1.**
- **CT/MRI pituitary fossa**: pituitary adenoma.

Complications
- **CXR**: cardiomegaly, **ECG**: ischaemia (DM and hypertension).
- **Pituitary function tests**: T_4, base line PRL and testosterone.
- **Glucose:** DM, **Ca^{++}**: MEN I.
- **Visual perimetry.**

Management

1 **Surgery:** trans-sphenoidal approach.
  Medical post-op complications
  - Meningitis.
  - Diabetes insipidis.
  - Panhypopituitarism.
2 **Medical therapy:** Cabergoline and Octreotide.
3 **Radiotherapy** in non-surgical candidates.

Follow-up

Annual GH, PRL, ECG, visual fields and CXR ± CT head.

MEN (multiple endocrine neoplasia) I

Inherited tumours: autosomal dominant, chromosome 11.
- **P**arathyroid hyperplasia ($Ca^{++} \uparrow$).
- **P**ituitary tumours.
- **P**ancreatic tumours (gastrinomas).

Causes of macroglossia

- **Acromegaly.**
- Amyloidosis.
- Hypothyroidism.
- Down's syndrome.

Acanthosis nigricans

- Brown 'velvet-like' skin change found commonly in the axillae.
- Associations:
  - Obesity.
  - Cultural: Indian subcontinent.
  - Type II diabetes mellitus.
  - **Acromegaly.**
  - Malignancy, e.g. gastric carcinoma and lymphoma.

Cushing's

Examine this lady and tell us what is wrong. She has been gaining weight.

Clinical signs: 'spot diagnosis'
- **Face:** moon-shaped, hirsute, with acne.
- **Skin:** bruised, thin, with purple striae.
- **Back:** 'buffalo hump'.
- **Abdomen:** centripetal obesity.
- **Legs:** wasting ('lemon on sticks' body shape) and oedema.

Extra points
- **Complications:**
  - **Hypertension** (BP).
  - **Diabetes mellitus** (random blood glucose).
  - **Osteoporosis** (kyphosis).
  - **Cellulitis.**
  - **Proximal myopathy** (stand from sitting).
- **Cause:**
  - **Exogenous:** signs of RA or asthma for example requiring steroids.
  - **Endogenous:** bitemporal hemianopia and pigmentation (if ACTH ↑).

Discussion
Cushing's disease: glucocorticoid excess due to ACTH secreting pituitary adenoma.
Cushing's syndrome: the physical signs of glucocorticoid excess.

Investigation
1 **Confirm high cortisol**
  - 24-h urinary collection.
  - Overnight dexamethasone suppression test.
2 **Low dose dexamethasone suppression test**
  - **Suppressed cortisol:** alcohol/depression/obesity ('pseudo Cushing's').
- **Not suppressed** → 3.
3 **High-dose dexamethasone suppression test**
  - **>50% suppressed cortisol:** Cushing's disease (60%).
    - **CT pituitary fossa** and **petrosal sinus vein sampling.**
  - **Not suppressed** → 4.

4 ACTH level
- **High:** Ectopic ACTH secreting tumour (15%).
  - **CXR.**
- **Low:** Adrenal adenoma (9%) or carcinoma (7%).
  - **CT abdomen.**

Treatment
Surgical: Trans-sphenoidal approach for pituitary tumours.
                 Removal of tumour.
- **Nelson's syndrome:** bilateral adrenalectomy (scars) to treat Cushing's disease, causing massive production of ACTH (and MSH), due to lack of feedback inhibition, leading to hyper-pigmentation and tumour growth.

Medical: Metyrapone.
              Radiation.

Prognosis
Untreated Cushing's syndrome has 50% mortality at 5 yrs (ischaemic heart disease due to diabetes and hypertension).

Causes of proximal myopathy
- **Inherited:**
  - Myotonic dystrophy.
  - Muscular dystrophy.
- **Endocrine:**
  - **Cushing's syndrome.**
  - Hyperparathyroidism.
  - Thyrotoxicosis.
  - Diabetic amyotrophy.
- **Inflammatory:**
  - Polymyositis.
  - Rheumatoid arthritis.
- **Metabolic:**
  - Osteomalacia.
- **Malignancy:**
  - Paraneoplastic.
  - Lambert–Eaton myasthenic syndrome.
- **Drugs:**
  - Alcohol.
  - Steroids.

Addison's

Examine this man, he was admitted as an emergency 4 days ago with hypotension.

Clinical signs
- Medic alert bracelet.
- Hyper-pigmentation: palmar creases, scars, nipples and buccal mucosa.
- Postural hypotension.

Extra points
- Other associated autoimmune diseases, e.g. hyperthyroidism, diabetes and vitiligo.
- Signs of TB or malignancy.

Discussion
Investigation order
1 **8 am cortisol** no morning elevation suggests Addison's disease (unreliable).
2 **Short Synacthen$^{®}$ test.**
  - **Exclude Addison's disease** if cortisol rises to adequate levels.
  - **If not → 3.**
3 **Long Synacthen$^{®}$ test.**
  - **Diagnose Addison's disease** if cortisol does not rise to adequate levels.

Other tests
Blood FBC: eosinophilia
U+E: ↓ Na^+ (kidney loss), ↑ K^+ ↑ urea (dehydration), ↓ glucose.
Autoantibodies.
CXR Malignancy or TB.

Treatment
Acute
- 0.9% saline IV rehydration + + +.
- Hydrocortisone.
- Treat the cause.
NB. 1 Anti-TB treatment increases the clearance of steroid therefore use higher doses.
  2 May unmask diabetes insipidus (cortisol is required to excrete a water load).

Chronic

- **Education:** compliance, increase dose if 'ill' (in bed), steroid card, Medic alert bracelet.
- Titrate hydrocortisone and fludrocortisone dose to levels/response.

Prognosis

- Normal life expectancy.
- In 80% of cases Addison's disease is due to an autoimmune process. Other causes include adrenal metastases, adrenal tuberculosis and Waterhouse–Friederichsen syndrome (meningococcal sepsis and adrenal infarction).
- Pigmentation is due to a lack of feedback inhibition by cortisol on the pituitary, leading to raised ACTH and MSH (melanocyte-stimulating hormone).

Appendix: Useful Addresses

Royal College of Physicians of London
11 St Andrews Place
London NW1 4LE
Tel: 020 7935 1174
Fax: 020 7486 4514
http://www.rcplondon.ac.uk

Royal College of Physicians of Edinburgh
9 Queen Street
Edinburgh EH2 1JQ
Tel: 0131 2257324
Fax: 0131 2252053
http://www.rcpe.ac.uk

Royal College of Physicians and Surgeons of Glasgow
242 St Vincent Street
Glasgow G2 5RJ
Tel: 0141 2216072
Fax: 0141 2483414
http://www.rcpsglasg.ac.uk

MRCP (UK) Central Office
11 St Andrews Place
London NW1 4LE
Tel: 020 7935 1174
Fax: 020 7486 4514
http://www.mrcpuk.org.uk

College publications:
MRCP (UK) Part 2 Clinical Examination (PACES) Clinical Guidelines.
MRCP (UK) Regulations and Information for Candidates:
• Guidance on examination structure and content.
• Examination mark sheets.

General Medical Council
178 Great Portland Street
London W1W 5JE
Tel: 020 7580 7642
Fax: 020 7915 3631
http://www.gmc-uk.org.

- Good medical practice.
- Guidance on confidentiality, consent and other ethical issues.

Index